JOHN ELKINGTON

THE POISONED WOMB

Human Reproduction in a Polluted World

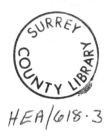

VIKING

VIKING

Penguin Books Ltd, Harmondsworth, Middlesex, England
Viking Penguin Inc., 40 West 23rd Street, New York, New York 10010, U.S.A.
Penguin Books Australia Ltd, Ringwood, Victoria, Australia
Penguin Books Canada Ltd, 2801 John Street, Markham, Ontario, Canada L 3 R 1 B 4
Penguin Books (N.Z.) Ltd, 182–190 Wairau Road, Auckland 10, New Zealand

First published 1985

Filmset in Monophoto Photina by
Northumberland Press Ltd, Gateshead,
Tyne and Wear

Printed in Great Britain by
Richard Clay (The Chaucer Press) Ltd,
Bungay, Suffolk.

Elkington, John
    The poisoned womb: human reproduction
    in a polluted world.
    1. Human embryo   2. Fetus—Diseases
    3. Pollution—Physiological effect
    I. Title
    618.3′2   RG627

ISBN 0–670–80110–0

To the Unborn

CONTENTS

PREFACE

This, even in such relatively relaxed times, is not a polite book. It focuses on most aspects of sexual reproduction, always a hazardous business but particularly so for those who have been exposed to radiation or to the growing list of chemicals known to affect sexual performance, fertility or the health of embryos, foetuses and surviving children.

It is not polite because it focuses on the experiences of ordinary people and on those whose carelessness or criminal negligence has caused sterility, apparently spontaneous abortions, birth defects or childhood cancers among those exposed. But, that said, my single objective has been to write a factually accurate, balanced account of an area of toxicology which is of growing concern both to the general public and to industry. *The Poisoned Womb* is a book about reproductive toxicology, but it is not simply a book for reproductive toxicologists. Today we all live on the toxic frontier and, in case after case, disaster after disaster, our reproductive systems have been showing the strain. The work of reproductive toxicologists is now of vital interest to us all.

Around the world, I have visited the laboratories of companies which are spending staggering sums of money to test the toxicity of their products, with no guarantee that unexpected side-effects will not still emerge once those products are in widespread use. Such companies often point to the context of the challenge they face in reproductive toxicology. The average mother and the average child, they say, are far safer and far healthier today than they were at the turn of the century – and the population statisticians agree.

As recently as 1900, for example, about fifty British women died in childbirth for every 10,000 live children born. And, in the early years of this century, about 100 children in every 1,000 live births died in their first year, usually in the first few weeks of life. Some countries, like Japan, have made astonishing strides since the Second World War in cutting maternal and infant mortality rates. But there has been a darker side to this near-miracle.

Better material living standards have typically brought better health, but they have generally been bought, particularly in the early years of an industrial economy, at the expense of widespread environmental pollution. Worse, as we all now know, some of the new materials developed by industry's synthetic chemists have proved to have a dramatic effect on sexual reproduction, whether in birds of prey or in people like us. And, as the Minamata disaster showed (pp. 23–4 and 32–4), even substances which have been in widespread industrial use over very long periods of time can still cause unexpected reproductive tragedies.

'Parts per *million* – just several millionths of something!' exclaimed the owners of the Chisso plant, which from 1956 devastated the lives of the fishing communities living along the shores of Minamata Bay. Now, we are routinely testing for chemicals at the parts per billion level, and some equipment can pick up chemical contaminants at the parts per quadrillion level. Even picking up one part per billion is equivalent to identifying one pea in a row of peas stretching from London to New York. Yet such astonishingly low concentrations of some chemicals can wreak havoc with sexual reproduction.

Anyone reading the papers or watching the television in recent years can hardly have missed the headlines about alleged links between chemical pollution and birth defects. In West Germany, Boehringer Ingelheim was forced to close a pesticide plant following fears that dioxin emissions had caused birth defects in nearby areas of Hamburg (p. 213). In Silicon Valley, several computer companies have been accused of causing miscarriages and birth defects (pp. 160, 211–13). And, in the United Kingdom, there was concern that two waste incineration plants operated by Re-Chem International might be responsible for yet more birth defects (p. 82).

Dr Alexander Speirs, a paediatrician who played a key role in identifying thalidomide as a teratogen, was warning that there should be a thorough scientific investigation of the children born with eye deformities near two toxic waste incineration plants in Wales and Scotland. Known as the 'Cyclops Children' by those living near the plant at Pontypool, the children had been born either with one eye or with tiny eyes, closed eyes or partial sight in one eye.

The company concerned, Re-Chem International, had just released a report commissioned from the Atomic Energy Research Establishment at Harwell, which appeared to show that levels of dioxin around the Scottish plant were normal for an industrialized country. As in many such cases, the evidence marshalled by industry's critics was largely circumstantial. Another problem is that the natural level of birth defects is relatively high. As the European Chemical Industry Ecology and Toxicology Centre has pointed out, the number of babies born with some sort of deformity is between two and three in every 100 births, with some of these defects only showing up years later. Many of these defects are caused by genetic disorders, some by environmental causes – including chemicals, drugs, infections or radiation. But how do you decide which of these causes is responsible for a particular deformity?

Spontaneous abortions, still-births and menstrual disorders were among the early effects reported in the wake of the worst-ever industrial disaster at Bhopal, in India. The release of the gas methyl isocyanate and, possibly, of cyanide, from the Union Carbide pesticide plant was reported to have resulted in over 2,000 deaths. As the death toll continued to mount, Union Carbide's manager of press relations described his state of mind as 'a continuous nightmare – only I wasn't asleep'. Inevitably, the nightmare had only just begun for many in Bhopal. Of the survivors, pregnant women were felt to be among the highest-risk groups.

The Poisoned Womb concentrates on three main types of threat: *carcinogens*, which can cause cancer, sometimes crossing the placental barrier to promote childhood cancers; *teratogens*, which can cause such effects as abortions, stillbirths, growth retardation, birth defects and longer-term behavioural changes in the affected children; and *mutagens*, which can damage our genes and chromosomes, possibly also triggering mutations.

It comes as a surprise to most people to learn that men are just as likely to have their reproductive systems disrupted by rogue chemistry as are women, although the effects differ between the sexes because of the fundamental differences in their reproductive systems. Imagine, for example, that Adam and Eve were both exposed to the same chemical in their post-Eden environment. Imagine, too, that this chemical caused chromosomal damage in those exposed to it. The reproductive toxicologist will tell you that such damage would be more likely to affect Adam if the exposure

happened when both he and Eve had reached adulthood. Sperm
production is a continuous process after puberty, and the repeated
cell divisions which take place during the sperm production cycle
afford endless opportunities for the chemical or other agent to
damage chromosomes.

Remove Adam from the chemical, however, and – provided that
his sperm-producing cells (stem cell spermatogonia) are not also
affected – his sperm production will pick up and the new sperm will
almost certainly be unaffected. Eve, on the other hand, could have
more of a problem, even if exposed during childhood. All the eggs
(ova) a woman will ever produce appear during the earliest stages
of her life, while she is still in her mother's womb (see p. 75). By
the time she is an adult, her ova are very much more resistant to
damage than are her partner's sperm. But if Eve had been exposed
during her early, vulnerable stages of development, and her ova
had been damaged, she would produce damaged ova throughout
her fertile life.

The Poisoned Womb discusses many other ways in which
chemicals and other agents can affect our reproductive systems. It
looks at the ways in which some of the more serious problems have
surfaced, at the tests which have been devised to identify the next
wave of potential problems, and at the regulatory dikes which have
been devised to sort out those chemicals likely to impose an unacceptable risk.

All risks are relative, of course: it is quite possible to poison
yourself simply by drinking pure water. As I wrote the final
sections of this book, a man, believing himself to have been
poisoned, unintentionally killed himself by taking no food and
attempting to flush out his system by drinking up to thirty-five
pints of water a day. The cause of death: water intoxication.

It is all too easy to succumb to paranoia when dealing with a
subject like reproductive toxicology, a point which a chemist with
Dow Chemical recently stressed when he said: 'If you are going
to say that one part per quadrillion of dioxin is dangerous, then we
are going to have to change our whole lifestyle.' He was joking,
and it is true that the increasing sensitivity of our analytical
equipment will soon mean that we shall be able to find every
known chemical in an ordinary glass of water. But if some of the
suspicions which are beginning to surface in reproductive toxicology are well founded, then we are going to have to retrace at
least some of our journey out from Eden.

ACKNOWLEDGEMENTS

Directly or indirectly, knowingly or unknowingly, many people have contributed to the shaping of this book. Anyone who attempts to understand and keep abreast of such a rapidly developing area of research must read a great deal and talk to a considerable number of people. I have done both. What follows is a highly selective listing of some of those who have helped, giving freely of their time, expertise and contacts.

Dr Michael Balls, director of the Fund for the Replacement of Animals in Medical Experiments (FRAME), Nottingham, helped me grapple with the complexities of traditional and emerging toxicity tests. Ronald Bayer, an associate of the Hastings Center, Hastings-on-Hudson, New York, brought me up to date on genetic screening research in the United States. Dr Rebecca Beaconsfield helped me to track down some of the work carried out on the human placenta by herself, her husband Professor Peter Beaconsfield and other members of the SCIP Research Unit at Bedford College, University of London. Shirley Liu Clayton of Genentech, Inc. showed me around the company's new animal testing facilities in south San Francisco. David Coleman of the Monitoring and Assessment Research Centre (MARC), London, alerted me to some of the sources used in Chapter I. Michael Dover, when at Penguin Books, helped with the early structuring of the book, while Tony Lacey of Viking and Alison Abel edited the final typescript. Mike Flux, group environment adviser at ICI, London, has helped me on a considerable number of points, as has Dr John Lawrence, director of ICI's Brixham Laboratory.

Dr Kenneth Harper, director of Life Science Research, helped with a briefing on the contract toxicology testing sector and with a tour of the company's facilities. Erik Jansson of Friends of the Earth, Washington, DC, gave me a great deal of very useful material on the Friends of the Earth campaign to get the US Congress thinking about reproductive hazards. Marek Mayer, as editor of the ENDS Report and long-time colleague at Environmental Data Services, London, has been a continuing source of up-to-the-minute information. Dr Richard Nicholson of the Society for the Study of Medical Ethics, London, helped with contacts and sources in a number of the areas covered.

Dr Clair Patterson of the Division of Geological and Planetary Sciences at the California Institute of Technology (Caltech) opened my eyes to some of the divergent views prevailing in the environmental monitoring community, and afforded me access to the results of his own pathfinding research. Dr Alan Pickaver of Greenpeace, Amsterdam, and Dr Brian Price of Friends of the Earth were instructive companions on a tour of Bayer AG's manufacturing facilities in West Germany.

Dr Alan Robertson, who was instrumental in founding ECETOC, explained some of the background to that organization's work in ecology, ecotoxicology and toxicology. Christopher Shorrock of Battelle ensured that I saw Battelle's new toxicology testing facility in Geneva. Sheila Silcock of the Royal Society for the Prevention of Cruelty to Animals provided me with a great deal of invaluable information on animal testing and related topics. Dr Andrew Sors was a valuable source of information on environmental monitoring during his time at MARC. Dr John Tesh of Life Science Research helped unravel the field of behavioural teratology. And Nigel Tuersley of the Earthlife Foundation provided some of the technical support needed in producing the book.

Anyone who wants to know more about reproductive toxicology would be well advised to track down a copy of *Reproductive Hazards of Industrial Chemicals* by Susan M. Barlow and Frank M. Sullivan of the Department of Pharmacology, Guy's Hospital Medical School, University of London. I found this book, published by the Academic Press in 1982, an invaluable reference work. Chapters 3 and 4 of *The Poisoned Womb* draw heavily on some of the cases reviewed by Barlow and Sullivan. Another splendid introduction to a component of this area of research, specifically mutagenicity testing, can be found in *Identifying and Estimating the Genetic Impact of Chemical Mutagens*, produced by the US Committee on Chemical Environmental Mutagens, the Board on Toxicology and Environmental Health Hazards, the Commission on Life Sciences and the National Research Council. Published by the National Academy Press in 1983, the book contains a wealth of information on the tests now being developed.

Some of the material used in this book has already appeared in *Biotechnology Bulletin*, the *ENDS Report*, the *Guardian*, the *ICI Magazine* and *Management Today*. I am grateful to these publications not only for allowing me to reproduce some of that information, but also for providing some of the resources which underwrote the research which produced *The Poisoned Womb*. I should also like to thank the Winston Churchill Memorial Trust. As a 1981 Churchill Fellow, I was able to visit a number of individuals and organizations in the United States at a critical time for environmental protection.

Finally, but by no means least, Elaine, Gaia and Hania have endured the lengthy gestation process and birth pangs which produced *The Poisoned Womb*. They have been unfailingly supportive, and had the book been on any other subject I should have dedicated it to them.

INTRODUCTION:
MOTHER-TO-BE

As the snow-capped bulk of Fuji-san, Japan's largest and most beautiful mountain, slipped by to the north and the *Shinkansen*, or bullet train, raced on towards Nagoya and Kyoto, my thoughts were several thousand miles away. Seen through the window of the speeding train, the snows of Mount Fuji had set me thinking of the flight over Greenland's icy wastes the previous month. Sitting in the window seat of the 747, I had been reading a report sent to me by Dr Clair Patterson of the California Institute of Technology, a report which gave me a totally different perspective on the astonishing scene sliding by below.

From horizon to horizon, the eye could pick out not a single trace of human habitation, let alone of industrial activity. Yet, Dr Patterson reported, core samples drilled from this Greenland ice and snow showed a twenty-fold increase in lead levels since the Industrial Revolution. Everywhere you go on this planet today, even in the trackless wastes of the polar ice-caps, you will find at least traces of pollution. Indeed, even the snows of Mount Fuji, floating above the gathering twilight and the very picture of purity, can be read as a litmus test of prevailing pollution levels.

Then, while my thoughts were still somewhere over Alaska, I woke up to the fact that a young Japanese woman had installed herself on the opposite bank of seats. Massively pregnant, she gazed out of the window of the *Shinkansen* at the flashing chimneys and unending factories of her country's sprawling industrial heartland.

Every so often she picked a strip of dried squid from one of the snack packs sold at any rail station and, as she did so, it hit me that here, in microcosm, was the theme of *The Poisoned Womb*.

A few months earlier, I recalled as the young woman turned from the window and lit a cigarette, an American paediatrician had published figures suggesting that the number of babies born with some physical or mental defect had doubled over the past twenty-five years. 'We're not seeing a very large increase in the number of children with flabby brains,' said Dr Peter Budetti, director of the Health Policy Program at the University of California, San Francisco, 'but there certainly is a big increase in the number of children with debilitating illnesses such as asthma and chronic bronchitis. Looked at another way,' he continued, 'compared with twenty-five years ago there are in the United States today at least half a million more children who have some limitation of activity due to either a chronic medical condition or a learning disability.'

As the mother-to-be puffed contentedly on her cigarette, sending smoke swirling up towards the ceiling of the compartment, I reviewed some of the explanations which had been put forward for this unprecedented rise in birth defects and other forms of infant ill-health. Some specialists are convinced that the rise is simply a product of our growing ability to diagnose congenital problems: the problems were there all along, they suggest, but we failed to spot them. Dr Budetti, by contrast, believed that there has been a real increase in the number of children born with defects. In the late 1950s, he argued, about 2 per cent of newborn babies had some physical, mental or learning defect, compared with about 4 per cent today. In Europe, meanwhile, between two or three of every hundred babies born are found to have some type of deformity. Among the suggested causes are increased smoking by women, increased exposure to a growing range of industrial chemicals, and medical progress which enables people with disabilities to survive and pass the disability on to successive generations.

Because environmental pollution is generally seen as a problem caused by *them* rather than us, by the greedy, remote industrialist squeezing every last cent out of his investment rather than by, say, the housewife driving to the supermarket, it is often blamed when other factors (some of them, like smoking, under our own direct control) are the real cause. But there is now indisputable evidence that a growing number of chemicals, many of which are found in the home, the workplace or the environment, can cause birth defects and an array of other reproductive problems. If the sole purpose of life is reproduction, as some biologists would have it, there are real grounds for believing that something, somewhere, has gone seriously wrong.

'Things just got so bad,' says one Japanese steel executive, describing the darker side of his country's economic miracle, 'that we finally realized that pollution didn't pay and that we'd eventually kill ourselves on these small islands.' As a result, almost a quarter of the money his company spends each year goes on pollution control equipment. You may still find that Mount Fuji is invisible from the window of your Tokyo hotel for days on end, because of the photochemical haze generated by that city's wall-to-wall traffic jams, but the yellow, sulphurous smogs which used to blanket the Tokyo–Osaka industrial conurbation ten years ago are, like London's smogs, largely a thing of the past.

Yet, even when such obvious problems have been rigorously controlled, the real environmental management problem has only just begun. The wastes that previously spewed out of factory chimneys and gushed from effluent outfalls have to go somewhere. A great deal can be done to redesign industrial production processes to ensure that they generate less pollution, but the conversion of raw materials into useful products always results in some degree of waste – and some of that waste is going to be toxic. In Japan, the Environmental Agency is responsible for controlling some 20,000 producers of toxic waste. These factories and other facilities generate about 1.5 billion pounds (0.68 billion kilograms) of toxic waste every year. While Japan's environmental regulations are now among the most stringent in the world, problems inevitably continue to surface.

And history is repeating itself in the new generation of economic miracle countries, such as South Korea and Taiwan. In Taipei, Taiwan's capital, the president of one American company based in the city advises joggers, 'Just breathe out.' Some days the air pollution is so thick that, as one local radio announcer has put it, 'you can hear pigeons cough and window washers can walk up to their jobs'. In the southern industrial city of Kaohsiung during 1982, for example, Taiwan's Bureau of Environmental Protection recorded up to 330 micrograms of lead, sulphate and other suspended particles per cubic metre of air. In Taipei, it found up to 186 micrograms per cubic metre, well in excess of the 'acceptable' standard of 140 micrograms set by the Bureau. For comparison, the relevant US standard at the time was 75 micrograms.

The Bureau, in fact, was set up only in 1982, but it was soon producing evidence of widespread health problems. These ranged from runny noses to cancer, with an unusually high level of childhood asthma found in cities like Taipei, and cancer, which can be caused by environmental pollution, replacing strokes as the leading cause of death in Taiwan. Even so, many Taiwanese believe that it will take at least another generation of economic development before the country will be willing to invest in really effective pollution control programmes. 'Only after reaching a certain stage in material lifestyle do people think of quality-of-life matters,' explained Professor Shih-chiao of the National Taiwan University.

Such problems cut right across political frontiers, as is forcefully illustrated by recent experience in Siberia. The rapid development of the region's natural resources has resulted in soaring birth-defect and worker-mortality rates, according to one Soviet scientist. 'First births are producing an increased number of defects and ailments,' said Professor Vlail Kaznacheyev, head of the Institute of Clinical and Experimental Medicine at the Siberian branch of the Academy of Sciences, 'and in this way we are transporting unhealthiness into the future.' These problems, he continued, were particularly acute in the south-west Siberian Kuznetsk Basin (or Kuzbass), an important area for coal and chemicals with a population of about 1.5 million. 'If we considered the Kuzbass as a giant plant producing health,' he concluded, 'then we would have to say it is turning out rubbish, irreparable rubbish. This is driving people away and causing an accumulation of genetic defects.'

Whether we live in Siberia, South Korea, Swaziland or Sweden, we all live on the toxic frontier. For those who live in the developing countries, caught up in the advancing surge tide of industrialization, life on the toxic frontier is in many respects an action replay of the environmental and health fallout which followed in the wake of our own Industrial Revolution. 'Only after they began giving birth to monsters did people wake up to the gravity of the problem,' said city councillor Dojival Santos of Cubatão, near São Paulo in south-eastern Brazil. Indeed, the plight of the 85,000 people living in Cubatão, which claims to be South America's largest industrial park, painfully illustrates the human impact of unchecked economic development.

It all began when Petrobrás, the government-owned oil mono-poly, built a refinery there in 1954. Hot on its heels came a rush of other companies, all eager to exploit the natural resources of the area and Brazil's largest market, São Paulo itself. Today, over twenty major factories discharge nearly a thousand tons of pollutants a day. Because of the local geography, easterly winds from the South Atlantic fail to clear the resulting pollution from the valley. In Vila Parisi, a *favela* or shanty town on the edge of the city, residents often suffer from a blotchy skin condition, known locally as 'alligator skin', caused by acid rain.

Even more strikingly, according to a study carried out by Pro-fessor Julio Groce of the Faculty of Medical Sciences in Santos, in 1982, almost 20 per cent of the *favela's* 15,000 residents had asthma, chronic bronchitis or rhinitis. He also found that over 35 per cent of all children over the age of five in Vila Parisi suffered from asthma, compared to an average rate around the world of perhaps 3 to 4 per cent. But far, far worse are the birth defects, which have been occurring in astonishing numbers. One of the most common is anencephaly, a partial or complete absence of the brain which is easily recognized because of the severely deformed skulls of its victims.

According to Romeu Magalhães, who claims that he was sacked from the local hospital when he threatened to make the facts about anencephaly known, 'It's an easy disease to verify, because the skull is soft and looks like it's been flattened by a gigantic hammer.' Dr Reinaldo Azoubel, Professor of Embryology at the University of São Paulo, has published strong evidence supporting the prosecu-tion case. 'The normal incidence of this disease is 1 case per 5,000 births,' he points out. 'Using data I gathered from Cubatão's death registry, however, the rate here was 1 case per 300 infants in 1982 and 1 case per 200 in 1981.'

A spokesman for Petrobrás, commenting on the health problems which are surfacing in the Cubatão area, has claimed: 'Malnutri-tion is the primary factor, and alcohol and smoking are also more important factors than our emissions. There has never been any corroboration that anencephaly is caused by industrial releases.' Sadly, today's comfortable consensus all too often, in retrospect, looks like yesterday's wanton neglect. 'How could the technical people in management, who should have known the risks, have allowed this to happen?' asks one Japanese worker whose work exposed him daily to hexavalent chromium for twenty-five years.

Taisuke Inoue's colleagues used to joke grimly that by the time they reached sixty-five they would be dying of lung cancer. Mr Inoue's respiratory tumours were diagnosed shortly before his sixty-fifth birthday.

Nutrition, alcohol consumption and smoking all have a significant impact on adult and foetal health. Research in Britain, for example, suggests that the poverty of some inner city areas may already be affecting the health of the unborn. Work carried out at the Nuffield Nutritional Laboratories suggests that the average baby born in affluent Hampstead, in London, is likely to be up to two pounds heavier than a baby born in a poorer area such as Hackney. It is thought that mothers who eat less than 1,700 calories a day during their pregnancy are significantly more likely to have retarded children, so the authorities recommend that mothers-to-be eat 2,100 calories a day during the first three months of pregnancy and 2,400 calories a day thereafter. A study of seventy-six women in Hackney revealed that they consumed an average of only 1,613 calories in the first three months of pregnancy, and 1,689 calories thereafter.

No one disputes that nutrition is important, and few people, even in Cubatão, dispute that those people in industrial employment are generally better fed than those who are unemployed or who exist outside the industrial economy. 'If I help force industry out of town,' said the father of two short-lived, deformed twins born in Vila Parisi, 'I lose my job. With no job, I can't feed my children, and they'll die a lot quicker from starvation than from pollution.' Or, as a local politician put it, his constituents 'do not prefer pollution to unemployment. They prefer neither, but they have been backed into a corner.'

It is all very well for a company like Petrobrás to plead that pollution is simply 'part of the price one pays for industry', but the question which a growing proportion of the world's population has been asking is: what price are we actually paying? Petrobrás, in fact, was responsible for the ensuing fireball which swept the Cubatão shanty town of Vila Socó early in 1984, killing an estimated 500 people, including some 300 children under the age of five (pp. 234–5).

Consider, too, the fish cancers which have been showing up in many areas of the world. In the Inner German Bight, for example, some 25 to 30 per cent of the fish caught are diseased, and environmental groups like Greenpeace have blamed the dumping of acid wastes there by West German chemical companies. In 1983, for the first time, the West German government admitted that there might be a relationship and called for the Commission of the European Communities to advance the date for the proposed banning of such dumping from 1993 to 1989.

In the United States, meanwhile, the problem was appearing in freshwater fish. A Congressional sub-committee was told that an 'epidemic of cancer' had hit fish as far apart as Seattle, on the west coast, and New York in the East. Fish collected from five sites across the country where human cancer rates were unusually high also showed exceedingly high cancer rates, said Dr John Harshbarger, director of the Smithsonian Institution's Registry of Tumors in Lower Animals. The five sites, all near major industrial centres, were: Puget Sound, in Washington State; Torch Lake, Michigan; the Black river in Ohio; and the Buffalo and Hudson rivers in New York State.

Liver cancers were found in Puget Sound English sole and starry flounder. Anyone who has walked along the Sound will know that it is an area of outstanding natural beauty, indeed my own daughters have spent many a happy hour playing along the water's edge there. But in some areas, it emerged, as many as one in four of the fish caught were affected by liver cancer. This figure could well have been higher, Harshbarger said, if early tumours were counted and fish too young to have developed tumours were dropped from the count. Surveys showed that, in some sites, such pollutants as aromatic hydrocarbons, polychlorinated biphenyls, chlorinated butadienes and heavy metals were present at levels perhaps thirty times those typically found in unpolluted areas.

In the Black and Buffalo rivers, liver and skin cancers were found in at least 30 per cent of the brown bullheads examined and the scientists found several dozen aromatic hydrocarbons in the river sediments, including a number of known carcinogens (cancer-causing agents). The picture at Torch Lake, however, was unique: liver cancers were found in *all* the sauger examined and in a large percentage of the walleyed pike. A leading cancer specialist, Dr John Black, has suggested that such fish cancers could be used as an alarm system by those concerned to prevent human health problems.

Fish, in fact, have been implicated in a number of major pollution incidents, such as the Minamata scandal. Indeed, had we been travelling through Japan seven or eight years earlier, that Japanese mother-to-be might have thought twice before buying her squid. Mercury-contaminated fish caused enormous suffering and many deaths in the fishing communities around Minamata Bay, with the result that many people stopped buying fish of any description. The Minamata poisonings took many in the medical profession by surprise because of the enormous damage done to some of the unborn children, children whose mothers showed few, if any, symptoms of mercury poisoning. Like a number of other toxic materials, mercury can cross the placenta and accumulate in the foetus.

Together with the thalidomide scandal, such pollution incidents gave a major boost to the emerging science of *teratology*, which involves the study of foetal development and of the ways in which its processes can be distorted by external agents such as drugs, environmental chemicals or radiation. Toxicology, as we shall see, has grown very rapidly indeed during the last decade, and reproductive toxicology, the subject of this book, has grown faster than most other areas of toxicology.

I confess I was surprised at how many of the Japanese companies we visited in Japan proudly showed us around their new reproductive toxicology laboratories. I was surprised for two reasons: first, I was leading a group of American and European biotechnologists around Japanese genetic engineering and biotechnology laboratories, so that reproductive toxicology was far from being uppermost in our minds; second, very few European companies would show visitors around their animal testing laboratories so freely because of sensitivities about animal rights. Even companies I have worked with over a number of years, like ICI, have kept me well away from their central toxicology laboratories, where chemicals and pharmaceuticals are tested on rodents and mammals.

Toxicity testing is a difficult business, a sensitive business, but very much a growth business. Yet even when the research results are in, there is no guarantee that the decision on whether to market the product is going to be cut-and-dried. It is impossible, as later chapters illustrate, to prove that a chemical product is safe. All it is really possible to say is that, used in a given dose in stated circumstances, it has not been shown to produce any side-effects or other problems. In some cases, however, there will be areas of uncertainty, of potential risk. The decision on whether to proceed will depend on how important the product is seen to be. Hoffman-La Roche, for example, warned druggists that Accutane, its prescription medication for acute acne, should not be used during pregnancy: three women using the product had recently delivered infants with deformities. If the risk had been one of cancer, the chances are that the product would have been withdrawn, although suspect birth control pills have stayed on the market, because the risk is either unproven or felt to be acceptable in the light of the risks run in conceiving and giving birth to a child.

There are four main classes of teratogen: radiation, viruses, drugs and chemicals. In this book we are mainly interested in chemicals and drugs, but the viral contribution is clearly important given that we have to tease out the effects of chemicals and drugs from background effects, and radiation is even more important, both because of its contribution to the background levels of cancers, birth defects and mutations, and because work on radiation biology underpins so much of today's reproductive toxicology.

Hiroshima was one of the cities I visited in Japan, and a great deal of research has been carried out on the impact of the atomic bombing there on the long-term health of the survivors. Surprisingly, given the very considerable numbers of people who suffered from radiation-induced disease, little or no evidence has emerged to suggest that the radiation has caused human mutations – which experiments with animals and insects had suggested were a strong possibility.

No one doubts that radiation can be deadly. Indeed, while I was in Hiroshima, the British nuclear power industry was in uproar because of accusations that the British Nuclear Fuels nuclear reprocessing plant at Sellafield (previously known as Windscale), Cumbria, had triggered a ten-fold rise in the local leukaemia rate. A Yorkshire Television documentary reported that plutonium dust had been found in local houses, and spot checks suggested that radiation levels in some local areas were 50 to 100 times higher than the natural background level. 'Leukaemia appears in clusters because it is rare,' cautioned Dr Alice Stewart, an expert on radiation risks based at Birmingham University. 'Common diseases usually spread evenly through the population. Rare ones appear as uneven outbreaks: it is a fact of statistics.'

The main problem in pinpointing the real cause of such 'hot spots' of disease is that the health effects of exposure to radiation are often expressed many years – and often decades – later. As Dr Stewart pointed out, 'These latest outbreaks could be the tip of an iceberg that will take a long time to melt away.' A few weeks later, further evidence emerged which suggested that radiation from a serious fire at the Windscale plant in 1957 had led to a sudden burst of cases of Down's Syndrome, or mongolism, on the east coast of Ireland. Six affected babies had been born to mothers who had all been teenagers at the same school in Dundalk when fallout from the accident, Britain's worst, reached the Irish coast. The babies, two boys and four girls, had been born between 1963 and 1972. According to Professor Irene Hillary of University College Dublin and Dr Patricia Sheenan, a consultant neurologist also based in Dublin, 'Irish meteorological reports are consistent with radio-active fallout having reached Ireland at a time of heavy rainfall in the Dundalk area. What happened to these young women when they were in school together? We are left with the nagging doubt that possible exposure to radiation associated with some infection had an adverse influence.'

'At the moment we do not know the most important fact in radiation biology,' commented Sir Douglas Black, the eminent physician appointed by the government to investigate the Cumbrian leukaemia hot spots. 'Is there or isn't there,' he asked, 'a safe level of radiation below which damage to people does not occur?' The report prepared by Sir Douglas and published in 1984 found 'no evidence of any general risk to health for children or adults living near Sellafield'. However, the Black report admitted that the incidence of leukaemia in nearby Seascale was roughly ten times the national average – and seven of the report's ten recom-mendations called for further research. Legislators would find it reassuring if they could be convinced that there is a 'no-effect' level of exposure to radiation or to a particular chemical, below which there is guaranteed to be absolutely no health effect. Sadly, how-ever, life is not quite like that. Constantly 'acceptable' levels of exposure, especially to chemicals, have had to be revised down-wards, and some scientists are convinced that there are effects right down the scale of exposure, with some people being more sensitive than others to such exposure.

Within days of the Windscale accusations having been aired, Cumbria County Council received a report from Professor John Fremlin, one of its advisers on radiological protection, concluding that the health hazards imposed by the levels of radioactive contamination found around the plant 'are trivial compared with the smoking of a single cigarette'. Then the ensuing inquiry, led by Sir Douglas Black, began to produce evidence that people under twenty-five living in the Millom rural district near Sellafield run a ten-fold greater risk of dying of leukaemia than does the average Briton in the same age-group. Who can blame the public for being confused about the risks to their health?

In fact, wherever science chooses to set a particular threshold of 'acceptable' exposure, public opinion may be mobilized against the source of radiation or chemical exposure long before the agreed threshold is breached. Industry has been increasingly aware of this fact. As we left Tokyo for a visit north of the city, for example, the news came through that a new crop of research findings had suggested that monosodium glutamate, the widely used flavour enhancer, could cause cancer. One of the biotechnologists on the study mission quipped that if the results of the tests in rats were accurate, 'we may have found the rat poison of the future'. More seriously, within hours a major manufacturer of monosodium glutamate, Ajinomoto, suffered a 10 per cent drop in the value of its shares. Although they recovered later, this near-miss illustrates the pressures such companies now operate under.

Walking around the toxicology laboratories run by such companies, with their sparkling new stainless-steel equipment and their shelves of violet-stained foetal dog and rat skeletons, it would be easy to dismiss them as little more than late twentieth-century versions of the witch's museum. A growing number of companies, however, see excellence in reproductive toxicology as a key element in the way they develop new products or seek new applications for their existing products. Meanwhile, the new toxicological and environmental analysis techniques can identify potential carcinogens, teratogens and mutagens at ever more rarefied levels, while the growing use of computers is enabling the medical profession to pinpoint relationships between exposure to such materials and even relatively small numbers of cases of disability, disease or death emerging at a later date.

In such circumstances, companies which want to stay in business really have no alternative. They are having to invest in toxicity testing laboratories and in staff recruitment and training, often moving ahead of the current regulatory requirements in the knowledge that regulations can be tightened overnight, leaving a whole business salient exposed and under fire.

It is still very much open to question whether the tests discussed in later chapters really do predict what is likely to happen in the real world, but for those with eyes to see, the writing is on the wall. If environmentalists and other pressure groups can convince a significant section of the public, or influential organs of the media, that a particular product or substance can affect the health of the unborn or of young children, as they have managed to do with lead in petrol, then industry's inability to prove a biological negative, to prove that a product or substance does not cause the alleged problems, can prove a fatal Achilles' heel. The ultimate decision is as likely to hinge on emotion and political horse-trading as on science. In the end, the unborn and our young children may get the benefit of the doubt.

Watching the young mother-to-be disappearing into the crowds at Kyoto station, it struck me that tracking her down several days later among the millions of people living in the vast Tokyo–Kyoto–Osaka conurbation would probably be easier than trying to monitor the environmental levels of some of the pollutants which could already have affected the long-term health of her unborn child. Some of these substances can represent a hazard even when present at the level of one part in a million, some at the parts per billion level.

In the last few years we have had to work out astonishingly accurate and sensitive techniques for measuring the levels of pollutants in materials as diverse as the snows of Mount Fuji, stuffed birds in museum collections, bat guano and Napoleon's wallpaper. Each of the many investigations described in later chapters would have taxed the powers of Sherlock Holmes to the limit. Of each he might reasonably have mused: 'It is quite a three-pipe problem.' Such problems are now part and parcel of life, disease and death along the constantly shifting toxic frontier.

ONE IN A
TRILLION

Read no further. Instead, tear a page from this book and send it to your nearest analytical chemistry laboratory – or pass it across to a friendly forensic scientist. Ask for a report on the levels of any chemicals not traditionally used in paper-making or in printing inks. Each page of every book published in the world today is, in effect, a litmus test of the environmental contamination levels prevailing where the original trees were grown, the wood pulped, the paper made, and the book printed and stored. And books have a particularly significant advantage if you are interested in pollution trends: they bear a publication date.

Take Japan as an example. Scientists in the chemistry department of Tokyo Metropolitan University built up a collection of books published between 1927 and 1972 and proceeded to treat them in a way which would give most university librarians palpitations. They opened each book in the middle, cut out about twenty pages (all of which were printed in black ink only), trimmed one centimetre of paper from the edge of each page, and cut the remainder of each page into strips. Five or six of these strips were then selected at random to represent each of the desecrated books.

Next, the sample paper was weighed and bathed in solvents, which were later distilled out of the mixture. This was then tested in a piece of equipment about which we shall be hearing more in the following pages: a gas chromatograph. What the scientists were looking for were residues of an organochlorine pesticide, hexachlorocyclohexane (or BHC), which had been widely used in Japan after its first introduction there in the mid-1940s.

Of all the organochlorine pesticides, BHC had been employed in the largest quantities in Japan, accounting for 90 per cent of the total volume used. The use of BHC peaked in 1968 with a reported figure of 46,830 tons – and stopped altogether, as far as the authorities were concerned, in 1970. But the persistent residues, scientists knew, remained in the environment and continued to migrate through it.

The sampling method used by the Japanese team, with only a few books sampled for each year, inevitably meant that the results gave a far from comprehensive picture of BHC contamination. As you might expect, the results from books published in the same year differed. But there was a very clear peak of contamination in 1946 and again, ten years later, in 1956. Interestingly, however, most of the books published *before* BHC was commercially used in Japan also proved to be contaminated to some extent, including those published in the late 1920s. These, it was concluded, had been contaminated at some point in their long shelf-life. No attempt was made to identify the pathways by which the BHC got into the more recently published books.

Indeed, anyone trying to analyse contamination in the products of today's paper industry faces a complex task. The industry uses more than 600 ingredients, including dyes, fillers, plasticizers, preservatives and whitening agents. Given that such chemicals as formaldehyde have been used, it is no surprise to find that those who work all day with certain types of paper have sometimes experienced unusual health problems. Doctors now talk of the 'secretary syndrome', the symptoms being rashes on the skin, drowsiness, headaches, and irritation of the eyes and lungs.

One woman who worked in the registrar's office at Pennsylvania State University, and had suffered from itchy rashes for about eighteen months, was referred to dermatologist Dr James G. Marks, Jr, at the University's Hershey Medical Research Center. He asked her to keep a log of the products she used and of the timing and duration of the rashes. The log provided convincing evidence that the problem was the colourless dye used in carbonless copy paper.

Another specialist who had diagnosed 'paper sickness' in a number of office workers was Professor Charles Calnan of the Royal Free Hospital, in London. A common feature of all the cases, Calnan said, was that, 'in the course of their work, they would frequently put a hand between sheaves of carbonless paper to extract a particular one, and they all noticed that this caused a tingling sensation of the skin.' But, he concluded, 'the evidence of an association of the symptoms described with the use of carbonless copy paper is entirely circumstantial and must remain supposition only. There is no proof.'

Tracking down conclusive evidence on types and sources of pollution can be a highly demanding task and, often, a politically fraught one. Consider the case of the mercury contamination found in Mediterranean tuna. The increasingly polluted Mediterranean was a fairly early target for the Global Environment Monitoring System (GEMS), set up in the wake of the 1972 United Nations Conference on the Human Environment, held in Stockholm. GEMS, which has justifiably complained that it is required to monitor the environmental health of an entire planet with 'a smaller budget than is enjoyed by the fire brigades of many large cities', set up a Mediterranean Pollution Monitoring and Research Programme to keep an eye on problems caused by such pollutants as oil, persistent insecticides and heavy metals. And the tuna, it found, were showing a high level of mercury contamination.

In the wake of the Minamata scandal, GEMS was taking no chances, particularly since tuna accounted for a significant proportion of the diets of many Mediterranean fishing communities. Mercury is a silvery, liquid metal which is about 13.6 times as dense as water. It is an excellent conductor of electricity and has therefore been widely used in electrical equipment, such as batteries, meters and switches, as well as in the electrolytic cells used to manufacture chlorine. But another major use, before 1971, was in the manufacture of biocides – from bacteriacides and fungicides through to antifouling and mildew-resistant paints.

Fortunately, the human body can take in and excrete as much as 2 milligrams of metallic or inorganic mercury a day without any sign of mercury poisoning. The symptoms of poisoning include tremors in the muscles and extremities. Anyone who has read Lewis Carroll's *Alice in Wonderland* will recall the Mad Hatter. If you made felt hats in the nineteenth century, you typically used a large quantity of mercury – and in hammering the felt into shape, you inevitably stirred up a fair amount of that mercury, which ended up in your lungs. As a result, many hatters developed incoherent speech, tremors and various mental disorders.

But far, far worse than inorganic mercury is organic mercury. The broadcasting of alkyl mercury substances, and particularly of methyl mercury compounds, was one of the gravest environmental misdemeanours of this troubled century. The two chemists who discovered diethyl mercury in 1865 paid for their success with their lives, and the whole family of organomercury compounds have proved to be dangerous poisons. And what science did not know until fairly recently was that several micro-organisms can produce the methyl mercury ion from any other form of mercury, metallic mercury included. Even the bacteria in the intestines of such birds as the common or garden hen proved able to produce methyl mercury. The most striking monuments to mercury poisoning can be found at Minamata Bay.

Over 120 adults and children living in a fishing village on Japan's Minamata Bay showed severe symptoms of what later came to be called 'Minamata disease', and forty-six of them died. A total of over 700 human poisonings were reported, with a 38 per cent mortality rate. As far as the infants and children were concerned, over twenty were born with or had soon developed a disease which in many respects was like infantile cerebral palsy – and the cause of all this suffering, which began in 1956, proved to be the methyl mercury released in effluents from the Chisso production plant. The plant, which manufactured chemicals, fertilizers, fibres and plastics, had used mercury as a catalyst in two processes: the manufacture of acetaldehyde (1932–68) and the production of vinyl chloride (1941–71). It has been estimated that the total losses of mercury to the aquatic environment from these operations were 81.3 tonnes and 0.2 tonnes respectively.

At first it was believed that the sole root of the problem had been the methylation of inorganic mercury by micro-organisms, fish and shellfish, the last two of which were an important element in the diet of the villagers. But measurements of the Chisso plant's effluents indicated that between 20 per cent and 40 per cent of the mercury discharged was probably discharged in an organic form. So Minamata Bay could have received about 30 tonnes of organic mercury by direct discharge.

Ultimately, the Japanese Ministry of Public Health and Welfare announced that the causative agent had been the methyl mercury compound contained in the effluent from the acetaldehyde plant. This is not to say that methylation in the environment played no part in the tragedy, but the results of studies of the mercury content of fish caught in the Bay were conclusive. Prior to 1966, when the Chisso plant ceased discharging these effluents into the Bay, the organic mercury content found in fish caught in the Bay ranged between 10 and 20 parts per million (ppm). After the discharges were halted, the concentrations did not exceed 0.5 ppm. Since the total mercury content of the sediments in the Bay did not presumably change during that period, the only explanation for this dramatic reduction in organic mercury levels must be that the effluents were the main source.

Methyl mercury causes severe mental retardation, seizures, loss of coordination in the voluntary muscles, partial or total loss of vision and hearing, and in severe cases it can also render its victims mute. It also has another unpleasant characteristic: it crosses the placental barrier. A pregnant woman eating mercury-contaminated fish endangers the health, indeed the life, of her unborn child – yet may show no symptoms herself.

The photographs of Japanese mothers cradling their crippled children seared their way around the world – and the GEMS findings suggested that the Mediterranean could well be next. Tuna are migratory fish, high up the food chain, concentrating the mercury absorbed or consumed by their prey. Industrial effluents, GEMS knew, are the most common source of mercury pollution. So, the experts concluded, 'somewhere around the Mediterranean, someone was contaminating the tuna's food sources', and it hoped that a careful survey would pinpoint the culprit.

But the first round of independently conducted surveys produced some confusing results. Each nation taking part found unusually high levels of mercury in its offshore waters – and many were reluctant to release their findings in case they were held responsible for mercury levels throughout the Mediterranean. Eventually, however, someone realized that all the participants were turning up high levels of mercury and a concerted attempt was launched to identify the source. In a matter of months the mercury was traced to low-level emissions from at least one submarine volcano in the eastern Mediterranean.

Industrial emissions, in short, might be responsible for some of the mercury contamination reported, but the overwhelming bulk appeared to come from natural rather than industrial sources. And in the United States mercury levels of 0.3–0.6 parts per million were found in tuna caught between 1878 and 1909 and subsequently preserved by the Smithsonian Institution. Mercury, to some degree at least, had been in the fish for decades. Effluents from factories like the Chisso plant may trigger localized catastrophes, but they are by no means the whole story.

Clearly, the ability to switch back to earlier periods of history and establish beyond doubt that particular environmental pollutants were either present or absent is a tremendous advantage – but, sadly, it is an ability we all too often lack. In some cases, the pollutants emitted have long since broken down and are now undetectable. With the advent of synthetic chemicals, however, we made sure that we left some fairly durable markers for many of our activities, including dish-washing. In Tokyo Bay another research team drawn from the Tokyo Metropolitan University and from the Geological Survey of Japan measured the amounts of alkyl benzene sulphonate (ABS) in Bay sediments. ABS was the active ingredient in many early synthetic detergents and the layering of sediments enabled the team to pinpoint years of peak use – between 1963 and 1975, when the concentrations of ABS were in the parts per billion range.

Unlike soaps, which are rapidly broken down by bacteria once discharged into the environment, ABS-based compounds have shown a surprising persistence. The scientists concluded that the ABS deposits found in sediments dating from the 1950s and 1960s had been largely unaffected by bacterial action. Later detergents, however, were designed to be biodegradable, breaking down fairly rapidly in the environment, so that there is a sharp decrease in the amount of ABS found in sediments dating from the 1970s.

Any material which builds up in layers can be used in this way, as long as there is some way in which the various layers can be dated and the layered material does not degrade the pollutant you are looking for. One of the stranger examples of this approach was reported in a scientific paper with the following, slightly mystifying title: *A Chronological Record of Environmental Chemicals from Analysis of Stratified Vertebrate Excretion Deposited in a Sheltered Environment.* In plain English, the paper was about the analysis of mercury levels in layers of bat guano found in a cave. The results gave a good idea of the trends in local pollution levels.

The idea behind the research was fairly ambitious. The two scientists involved, Michael Petit and Scott Altenbach, knew that an unexpectedly high proportion of environmental mercury could be coming from natural out-gassing of the Earth's crust and upper mantle. If so, they argued, then we might expect major periods of glaciation to have significantly influenced the amount of mercury in the atmosphere. They suggested that one way of checking this idea would be to work through the annual layers of guano in caves used by the migratory free-tailed bat, *Tadarida brasiliensis*, to see how mercury levels changed over time. Using radio-carbon dating techniques, one guano deposit in the Carlsbad Caverns National Park had been shown to be over 17,800 years old.

To test their idea, they picked a bat cave near Morenci, Arizona, which had previously been mined down to bedrock – so that they could establish the exact age of the deepest layer of guano. And the question they specifically set out to answer was whether changing levels of atmospheric pollution could be tracked accurately in the successive annual layers of bat guano. They took core samples from the guano in a cave located some 5.25 miles, as the crow flies, from a large copper smelter and open-cast mine. When the samples had been agitated in a digesting solution for forty-eight hours, they were analysed by cold-vapour atomic absorption, using a double-beam mercury analyser – and the results are crystal clear.

There is a remarkably close fit between the trend line representing mercury contamination in the bat guano and the trend line representing levels of copper production at the smelter. The two marked slumps in copper production, during major strikes at the plant in 1957–9 and 1967, are clearly reflected in the two large decreases identified in the guano deposits for 1958 and 1968 in Eagle Creek cave. Interestingly, there is a one-year delay between changes in copper production and the related change in mercury levels in the guano – which suggests that the mercury did not enter the bat food-chain through the adult moths which form the bulk of the bat diet. Instead, it seems, it entered by way of vegetation eaten by the moth larvae some time before they reached their adult stage.

Many other materials have been analysed during research into historic levels of environmental contamination, including tree-rings, preserved animal and plant materials held in museum collections or herbariums, human bones, teeth, nails and hair. There are serious problems with interpreting the results from many of these materials. To be really useful, the material must have a number of characteristics: it must be able to retain a pollutant for a period of time; it must absorb the relevant pollutant at a defined rate; it must allow dating, although not necessarily as accurately as a book or bat guano; and there must be enough of the material to permit adequate statistical analysis.

Tree-rings can sometimes echo changes in local contamination caused by factories or road traffic, but most of those who have used what is called 'dendroanalysis' have found it far from infallible. Feathers, too, have limitations: they reflect the contamination prevailing during only a short period of moulting, not during the bird's entire life. None the less, Swedish investigators found roughly constant mercury levels in the feathers of preserved birds from 1840 to 1940, followed by a distinct increase in the 1940s and 1950s – when many countries were using methyl mercury in seed dressings. Dramatic drops in bird populations, and particularly of predatory birds, were observed. In most cases, the eventual banning of such seed dressings resulted in the populations of both seed-eaters and predators rebounding.

Human hair is the last material we shall consider here. Roman hair excavated near Dorchester has given an impression of environmental conditions as long as 2,000 years ago. Mercury and arsenic analyses have been carried out on the hair of a number of suspected poisoning victims, including King Charles II of England, whose enthusiasm for alchemy may have led to the high levels of mercury found in his hair, and Napoleon Bonaparte. Hair has been found to be an accurate indicator of some metal contaminants, such as arsenic, cadmium and lead, but not of others, including copper and zinc.

The story of Napoleon's death, now sufficiently far in the past to be a great deal less politically sensitive than, say, the levels of mercury in the flesh of Mediterranean tuna, provides a fascinating illustration of some of the technologies now used to measure very low concentrations of particular contaminants. And, given that we began by looking at contaminants in various types of paper, it is interesting to note that Napoleon may have succumbed to poisoning from a totally unexpected quarter: his wallpaper.

As with so many of the other poisonings discussed in these pages, this particular episode was only brought to light because it attracted the attention of someone with the instincts of a detective. Dr David Jones first became interested in a copper arsenite pigment called 'Scheele's green' when he was researching a light-hearted talk for BBC Radio Scotland. He was particularly interested in the poisoning of many hundreds of householders during the nineteenth century. The Swedish chemist Scheele had discovered the pigment in 1775, and it had been used in an increasingly wide range of paints, fabrics and wallpapers. Then, slowly, it had become clear that the arsenic in the new pigment could escape from such materials and find its way into the human body.

Next, in 1893, an Italian biochemist discovered that the problem arose only when the green wallpaper became damp and mouldy. If a mould, such as *Scopulariopsis bevicaulis*, is to survive in such a toxic environment, it has to have some way of getting rid of the arsenic – and, it turned out, a number of them did. They converted the arsenic into vapour, or arsenic trimethyl, and discharged it into the room, where the occupants duly breathed it in.

All this reminded Dr Jones of the discovery, by means of neutron-activation analysis, that surviving samples of Napoleon's hair contained suspicious amounts of arsenic. Exiled to the South Atlantic island of St Helena after his final defeat at Waterloo, Napoleon was housed from his arrival in October 1815 to his death in May 1821 in a wooden building, Longwood House, which was apparently chronically damp. Napoleon suffered from a number of symptoms during his stay on the island, including shivering, sicknesses, diarrhoea, stomach pains and weaknesses and swellings of the limbs. Interestingly, however, many of his companions also suffered from illnesses of this sort – 'just what you would expect,' Dr Jones concluded, 'if the basic cause were not deliberate poisoning at all, but arsenical wallpaper'.

Now came the difficult part of the exercise: how to establish whether Longwood House was actually decorated with the right sort of green paint or wallpaper. When his radio talk was broadcast, Dr Jones included, 'purely as a cheerful throwaway line', the following question: 'If any historian listening can tell me, I'd be fascinated to know – were Napoleon's rooms or dungeons or whatever on St Helena decorated with green paint or wallpaper?'

Then, in what Dr Jones described as 'the most astonishing piece of scientific good fortune of my life', he received a letter from a woman in Norfolk who reported that she had a common-place book, dated 1823–9, in which there was a sample of wallpaper with the following words beside it: 'This small piece of paper was taken off the wall of the room in which the spirit of Napoleon returned to God who gave it.' She sent him the wallpaper specimen, which was about six centimetres square, and his producer promptly rang Glasgow University, where the original analysis of Napoleon's hair had been performed. He reported back that Dr Ken Ledingham, a physicist with the University's Kelvin Laboratory at East Kilbride, would be willing to examine the sample by X-ray fluorescence spectroscopy.

This technique involves bombarding a sample with high-energy radiation. When this hits an atom, it triggers changes in the position of electrons in the atom's electron shells which, in turn, result in the emission of X-rays. Since each element emits a characteristic fluorescent X-ray, the resulting spectra can be readily interpreted. And the very first spectrum produced at the Kelvin Laboratory showed arsenic. Later, however, it became clear that the whole book contained arsenic, which was apparently a common contaminant of nineteenth-century paper. So they detached the wallpaper from the page and proceeded to examine it separately.

Confusingly, the wallpaper's central rosette, where the arsenic seemed to be concentrated, also had a lot of lead in it. This caused a number of problems: lead absorbs X-rays, resulting in false spectra: one of lead's fluorescence peaks overlaps the arsenic peak, obscuring it; and they found irradiation of the paper gave different results, depending on which face was uppermost. A further problem surfaced when it was realized that the calibration papers bought by Dr Jones were inconsistent. This paper, doped with known amounts of arsenic or whatever other material is of interest, is used in the spectroscopy work to calibrate the equipment.

At last, with new calibration papers prepared, Dr Ledingham was able to disentangle the problem, screening out the interference generated by the layers of lead in the sample – and the conclusion was that the central rosette, whose green decoration was thought to be copper arsenite, contained 1.5 grams per square metre of arsenic. Using a photograph of replica wallpaper, the average arsenic content of Napoleon's wallpaper was estimated to be about 0.12 grams per square metre.

But, Dr Jones was then forced to ask, was this a sufficiently toxic arsenical wallpaper to have produced the recorded health effects? Samples of arsenical wallpaper from an historic house in Northumberland had produced readings of 6 grams per square metre, fifty times more toxic than Napoleon's wallpaper, which, as Dr

Jones put it, 'looked positively anaemic by contrast'. He persevered, however, embarking on a long, tedious search through the Victorian medical literature for reliable analyses of toxic arsenical wallpapers. Most of the accounts he was able to track down were vague in the extreme, but ultimately he found a paper published in 1893 which analysed twenty cases of wallpaper poisoning. The wallpapers contained between 0.015 and 0.6 grams per square metre – a range which extended well below the level found in Napoleon's possibly deadly decor.

The author of that paper, a Dr Sanger, also suggested that these less arsenical papers could well prove more toxic, since mould could proliferate on them much more readily than on highly arsenical papers. Just to clinch matters, it was decided to use a different analytical technique: neutron activation analysis, the same technique that had been used by the Swedish investigators when testing bird feathers for mercury.

This technique works as follows. Many elements undergo nuclear reactions when exposed to a strong neutron-flux in a reactor, being converted into specific short-lived radio-isotopes. These isotopes are so radioactive that even very small amounts of the original elements, measured in nanograms, can generate detectable radioactivity. Using a solid-state detector and spectrometer system, as used in X-ray fluorescence, it is then possible to establish from which elements the isotopes came. Arsenic, fortunately, is fairly readily activated in the reactor and is detectable in amounts as low as a few parts per million – which explains how it was possible to analyse Napoleon's surviving hair.

The overall conclusion: the arsenical wallpaper almost certainly did not kill Napoleon, but it probably did contribute to his illnesses – and may well account for the arsenic found in his hair. This tortuous detective story, meanwhile, has prepared the ground for a discussion of one of the bedrock facts of life which toxicologists and polluters alike must now recognize: our latest analytical technology can sense the presence of contaminants at levels which even a few years ago would have been unthinkably low.

'Parts per *million* – just several millionths of something,' the directors of the Chisso plant exclaimed when they were accused of poisoning the waters of Minamata Bay. They also pointed out that, at the time of the discharges, equipment able to measure such concentrations of mercury simply did not exist. But by 1975 mercury poisoning had been confirmed in 798 people and was suspected in a further 2,800. The company was forced to pay indemnities exceeding $80 million, with more to come. 'A million or two invested in environmental research and monitoring,' GEMS commented later, 'when fish were first found floating dead in Minamata Bay, when cats went mad and when people began to develop symptoms of a strange disease, would have been much cheaper and infinitely more responsible. But the cruel truth is that almost to the end lack of scientific evidence could stand as a secure defence for inaction.'

Consider, however, what one part in a million actually means. One part per million (ppm) equals one milligram per kilogram of the material which has been contaminated – or, to put it another way, one ppm is roughly equivalent to one drop of water out of 16.5 gallons. It is equivalent to one minute in two years. And some of the new equipment can now sense contaminants at the parts per billion (ppb), trillion or quadrillion level. Some pollutants are dangerous even at ppb levels, yet one ppb is a drop of water in a swimming pool measuring 3m × 3m × 6m. It is one minute in 2,000 years. Dow Chemical is one of the companies which can now operate at the parts per quadrillion level.

The use of gas chromatographs has pushed back the analytical frontiers to an astonishing extent. Gas chromatography is a technique used to separate mixtures of volatile substances, such as chlorinated hydrocarbons. The sample to be analysed is placed on a separating column and is washed through with an inert gas. The column then selectively retards (and thus separates) the substances contained in the mixture. The column material is usually coated with a relatively non-volatile liquid, called the 'stationary phase', which gives rise to the term gas–liquid chromatography.

The fact that some laboratories can now measure the equivalent of one pea in a row of peas from London to New York, however, does not mean that there are no disputes between laboratories about what is or is not present in particular samples. Far from it. Take the lead issue as an example. One of the severest critics of the current state of lead research has been Dr Clair Patterson of the California Institute of Technology (Caltech). Dr Patterson's analytical equipment is so sensitive and accurate that he believes he has pinpointed massive errors in the reported findings of many other lead researchers.

The specific question he has been addressing is this: how much more lead are we exposed to today, from all sources, than were our ancestors several thousand years ago? Dr Patterson stresses that the results achieved by investigators when dealing with highly contaminated samples from urban areas and with the blood of lead-poisoned people are often accurate. The industrial lead found in such samples exceeds some 10,000-fold the naturally occurring lead they contain, so reasonable precautions taken during sampling, handling and analysis can cut out large positive errors. But the situation is altogether different where measurements are being taken of natural lead in the environment.

If we assume that the natural level of lead in a remote region, lead which has been weathered from rocks and then found its way into water, plants and animals, is accurately analysed as 10 units in a given sample, then Dr Patterson suggests that roughly 100 units will have been added by the long-distance transport of lead from road traffic and industrial sources – and an astounding 500 units will have been introduced into the sample by the investigator himself during the sampling procedure. And, as though that were not enough, he has calculated that a further 500 units can be added during poorly controlled analysis in the laboratory.

'Most investigators fail to properly reduce or subtract this lead they add to the samples they have collected,' he says. Investigators entering remote regions, he points out, 'bring with them from heavily polluted urban regions such large quantities of industrial lead adhering to their equipment, bodies, life support systems and transport that improperly controlled transfer of tiny fractions of this intruded lead to collected samples of materials completely overwhelms the sums of natural and environmentally added industrial lead already in the materials.'

As they drive or fly back to their laboratories, many such investigators 'have no idea of the proportion between the natural lead and the environmentally added industrial lead originally in the samples. They bring this undefined mixture of three different kinds of lead in samples back to their extremely polluted urban laboratories. Then, swimming in pools of industrial lead, they tend to make blind, incorrect and insufficient subtractions for lead blanks supposedly added to their sample during analyses.'

The end result is that most lead investigators severely over-estimate contamination in such remote regions. The table compares lead concentrations reported in the scientific literature with the results achieved at Caltech. 'Our data derive from isotope dilution mass spectroscopy,' Dr Patterson explains, 'used under ultra-clean laboratory conditions, a technique that I developed. This is a very powerful and accurate analytical method for trace amounts of lead. However, it is extremely cumbersome, very costly and very time-consuming: as a consequence, it can generate only relatively small amounts of data.' One can see why many laboratories opt for cheaper, less accurate alternatives.

Comparisons between actual and commonly reported lead concentrations (source: Caltech)

Material	Actual concentration determined at Caltech	Reported concentration in the literature
ultra pure laboratory water	100–500 femtograms Pb/g	100–1,000 picograms Pb/g
old glacial ice	1 picogram Pb/g	50–5,000 picograms Pb/g
deep sea water	1–6 picograms Pb/g	500–10,000 picograms Pb/g
remote fresh water	5–50 picograms Pb/g	500–10,000 picograms Pb/g
human blood plasma	0.1 nanograms Pb/g	30–300 nanograms Pb/g
marine fish muscle	0.3–0.4 nanograms Pb/g	300–800 nanograms Pb/g
remote tree trunks	1–3 nanograms Pb/g	1,000–10,000 nanograms Pb/g

Notes: Lead (Pb) levels are reported in grams (g), nanograms (10^{-9}g), picograms (10^{-12}g) and femtograms (10^{-15}g).

A common characteristic of the laboratories which Dr Patterson allows *are* accurate, including a laboratory at the University of Paris and another in Denver, Colorado, is that they are capable of carrying out reliable studies of lead in lunar rocks or in very exotic cosmological debris. The costs of the US facilities have to a considerable extent been underwritten by the US space effort.

The immediate assumption on reading all this might be that lead pollution problems have been exaggerated: not so. Indeed, the more accurate measurements now available from Caltech suggest the reverse. Industrial lead emissions, says Dr Patterson, 'have been so excessive in relation to natural occurrences of lead that most people living with industrialized societies contain 500 to 1,000 times more lead in their bodies than did their prehistoric ancestors. The extent of this exposure is so great that it is highly probable that most people are suffering ill effects from it. The identification of the exact nature of these ill effects, however, poses formidable problems, since no suitable control populations exist in the modern world.'

The use of control populations in environmental medicine will be explained in more detail in Chapter 4, but the central problem here is that the groups of adults and children used to establish a baseline against which poisoning in 'exposed' groups can be assessed are themselves exposed to about 500 times more lead than were their ancestors. Figure 1.1 compares the relative lead levels found in people at different times in history. The natural amount found in prehistoric peoples is illustrated on the left with a single dot, with each dot representing 0.0003 grams in a 70-kilogram person (expressed scientifically as 3×10^{-4}g Pb/70-kg person). The middle figure represents the average present-day American, shown with 500 dots. And the third, right-hand figure, speckled

Fig 1·1

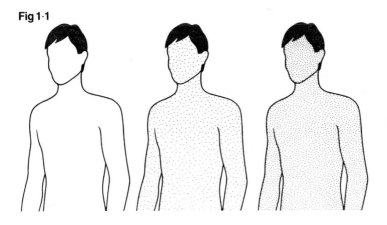

Figure 1.1   A comparison of the relative amounts of lead in people at different points in history. Each dot represents a unit of lead equivalent to 3×10^{-4}g Pb/70 kg person (see above for explanation). The left-hand figure depicts the natural amount in prehistoric man (one dot). The central figure shows the average amount in present-day man living in an industrialized region (500 dots). The right-hand figure shows the minimum amount (2,000 dots) at which a significant proportion of those exposed will show symptoms of classical lead poisoning. (*Source*: Patterson, Caltech)

with 2,000 dots, shows the minimum level of contamination needed to cause classical lead poisoning in a significant number of people.

It is now clear why Dr Patterson's new analytical methods are so important. The contrast between the body lead burdens of the left-hand and central figures was not discovered until recently, largely because the ubiquity of industrial lead has made it, in some respects, 'invisible' to many investigators, because it now constitutes a constant background feature. Living representatives of the left-hand figure have not been observed, but careful research on prehistoric human skeletons and food-chains has shown, for example, that Peruvian Indians living some 2,000 years ago had body lead burdens which were less than one-thousandth of those measured in today's North Americans.

So some investigators have been 'blinded' to the real lead problem in very much the same way that the lead layers in Napoleon's wallpaper blinded the analytical equipment to the presence of significant concentrations of other contaminants. The only way to ensure real comparisons between lead-free and lead-poisoned animals or people, Dr Patterson has suggested, would be to build lead-free laboratory sanctuaries. But this would be 'an inordinately difficult task', partly because the analytical equipment available to date could not guarantee lead-free nutrition for the animals.

According to the UN about 500,000 of the millions of chemical substances known are now in use, with about 10,000 produced in quantities of up to 1,000 tonnes. The US National Academy of Sciences believes that some 70,000 synthetic chemicals are used and traded in the United States, of which perhaps 25,000 are in 'common use'. In addition, between 700 and 3,000 new chemicals are introduced each year. The National Academy of Sciences feels that it is reasonable to assume that the US population may be exposed to at least 50,000 chemicals. Few of these chemicals are as widely dispersed in the environment as is lead, but their novelty has meant that the regulatory authorities have too often been taken by surprise by the emergence of totally unexpected ecological and human health problems.

Indeed, there are those in the medical profession, dubbed 'clinical ecologists', who see the emergence of what has been called 'total allergy syndrome' as a warning that our immune systems are failing to keep pace with the chemical environment we are producing for ourselves. One *cause célèbre* in the early 1980s was the case of Sheila Rossall, the former pop singer who was described as being 'allergic to the twentieth century'.

By 1981, her health had deteriorated to such an extent that she weighed only 24.5 kilograms and found it much easier to list the substances she was not allergic to than those to which she reacted. These were cotton, hardwood, silk, stone and stainless steel. Almost any other material irritated her body intensely and, in some cases, triggered convulsions very much like those experienced in epilepsy. When she was flown from Britain to Dallas, the entire plane's heating system had to be switched off to allow the plastic pipes used to give her oxygen to cool down and stop giving off the fumes which had twice pushed her into unconsciousness during the flight.

She was being taken to the Environmental Unit at Brookhaven Hospital, where patients with intense allergies to our ubiquitous industrial chemicals are effectively insulated against the twentieth century. Double doors, rooms lined with such inert materials as tiles or aluminium, stone floors, metal furniture, pure cotton curtains and filters which pass air over activated charcoal to remove stray chemicals: all these and more are to be found at the Brookhaven unit. Notices abound, with such messages as 'Do not enter this area if you are wearing perfume, hair-spray or after-shave lotion'.

The unit was set up by Dr William Rea, who had himself developed a severe allergy syndrome when his home was sprayed with a pesticide – after which he became sensitive to anaesthetic gas and to chemicals used in heart-lung machines, basic tools of his trade. He subsequently began to develop the ideas of Dr Theron Randolph, known as the father of clinical ecology. Supporters of this approach argue that the scale of chemical adulteration of today's processed foodstuffs is scandalous, pointing to the widespread use of such chemicals as butylated hydroxy anisole, butylated hydroxy toluene, monosodium glutamate, nitrate, sodium benzoate or tartrazine, all of which can cause reactions in those sensitive to them.

Clinical ecology has not been without its critics, some of whom have proved to have a 'total allergy reaction' to the whole concept of total allergy syndrome. 'Some anxious people are very suggestible, and when told that they are sensitive to chemicals in the environment are inclined to believe it,' said one leading British allergy expert, Professor Jack Pepys. 'The consequences for their life may then be disastrous because they spend all their time avoiding imaginary dangers. Medical advice given without definite proof is very dangerous because it can create a psychoneurosis.'

Allergies to such twentieth-century materials as cleaning agents, glues, paints or plastic foams, such experts accept as fairly common, but they are distinctly unhappy when it comes to claims that patients may become sensitized not just to one substance, but to a wide range of substances. Clinical ecologists like Professor Doris Rapp, however, insist that the problem is real, is growing and needs to be dealt with promptly. 'A growing number of young people are totally incapacitated because of pollution in the air, the water, our homes and our food,' she argues. 'Doctors must face up to it. We can't sit on our hands and say nothing is happening.'

If the clinical ecologists are even partially correct in their conclusions, then the implications for the medical profession and, more particularly, for the chemical industry will be enormous. But what is clear, meanwhile, is that some elements of our chemical environment are causing increasingly significant human health problems, many of which are producing symptoms which are taxing the skills and resources of toxicology to the limit.

'For the first time in the history of the world,' Rachel Carson wrote in *Silent Spring*, 'every human being is now subjected to contact with dangerous chemicals, from the moment of conception until death.' Toxic metallic compounds, including those based on arsenic, lead and mercury, have been recognized as a threat to human health for many decades. As we shall see in later chapters, they still constitute a grave threat to ecological stability and to human health: each year, for example, 13,000 tonnes of metal go down Britain's drains in industrial effluents, the equivalent of four small warships. But if these materials are toxic, many synthetic chemicals are considerably more so.

Rachel Carson was particularly concerned about the 'enormous biological potency' of the new synthetic insecticides – or biocides, as she preferred to call them. 'They have immense power not merely to poison but to enter into the most vital processes of the body and change them in sinister and often deadly ways,' she warned. She marshalled evidence from all over the world to prove conclusively that chlorinated hydrocarbons and organic phosphorous insecticides were responsible not only for killing wildlife, but also for interfering with animal reproduction – an activity which many evolutionary biologists define as *the* most vital process of the body.

Before we focus on those 'unborn canaries', the world's human embryos and foetuses (see, p. 65) and lest the reader assume that reproductive toxicology is exclusively a concern for mothers or potential mothers, consider what has been happening to some fathers – or would-be fathers. If the peregrine falcon and the bald-headed eagle were the unwitting symbols of the poisoning of wildlife by synthetic crop protection chemicals, it is fair to say that the human sperm is in danger of becoming, along with the human egg and embryo, their symbolic counterpart as far as the chemical disruption of the human reproductive cycle is concerned.

CHAPTER TWO

THE
ENDANGERED
SPERM

And now, they say, even sleep can damage your health and, possibly, the health of future generations. Human sperm counts have been falling for some time in industrialized countries such as the United States, some research results suggesting that the average American male today produces less than half of the sperm produced by the average male some fifty years ago. One possible cause, suggested by Dr Ralph Dougherty of Florida State University, is the use of foam mattresses. When he ran tests on semen donated by students he found traces of Fyrol FR2, a flame-retardant used to cut down the fire risks associated with foam-filled furniture.

Around the world, scientists have been reporting unexpectedly high concentrations of such chemicals as polychlorinated biphenyls (PCBs) in semen samples. Such chemicals, widely disseminated in the environment by various industrial activities, are increasingly seen as likely culprits for the parallel downward trend in reported sperm densities, although there are a number of possible confounding factors. Sperm density and male fertility can be reduced, for example, by increased sexual activity, by smoking, by drug abuse and by alcoholism. They are also influenced by temperature: men who live in colder climates tend to show higher sperm counts, as do men who wear loose-fitting underwear which affords easy air circulation around the groin, cooling the testicles.

But, even allowing for these factors, there is strong evidence that the increasing exposure of modern man to a growing number of industrial chemicals is producing measurable drops in male fertility leading, in some cases, to actual sterility. When Dr Dougherty sat down to analyse his findings, it turned out that 23 per cent of the male students tested at Florida State University were functionally sterile – showing less than twenty million sperm cells in each millilitre of semen. These low sperm counts are an indication that some American males now produce *less than a quarter* of the sperm produced by the average American half a century ago. Functional sterility does not imply a total inability to father children, but it can result in considerable difficulties being experienced by would-be fathers. Combined with those of other studies, Dr Dougherty's results suggested that by the 1980s some 20 per cent of American males could be functionally sterile, compared with only 0.5 per cent in 1938, when scientifically sound sperm counts began.

Not surprisingly, these results were soon picked up by environmental groups such as Friends of the Earth. In the United States, Friends of the Earth wrote to all members of Congress with a package of information culled from the scientific literature which, they argued, showed that 80 per cent of all birth defects now reported in the United States derive from the male parent – and that the sharp drop in sperm counts, particularly since the 1960s, appears to be a major factor affecting these high birth-defect rates, with chromosome aberrations increasing significantly when sperm counts are low.

Paradoxically, one result of the decline in sperm counts has been a growing use of artificial insemination which has, in turn, highlighted the contribution defective sperm can make to birth-defect rates. For readily understandable reasons, artificial insemination clinics use third party donors with high sperm counts, and the result is that birth defects resulting from artificial insemination are very low – typically less than 1 per cent, compared with expected rates of 4–6 per cent. Clearly, such clinics will also tend to screen their donors for possible congenital problems, but Friends of the Earth were convinced that 'American men presently cause the vast majority of birth defects and sperm counts are the major variable in birth defects'.

Among the chemicals Dr Dougherty found in the semen samples were PCBs, Fyrol FR2 and three kinds of polychlorophenols, a family of chemicals used as insecticides and fungicides. 'The levels are in the order of parts per billion,' said Dr Dougherty, 'and that's not really much. But it is enough to cause measurable biological effects.' He saw his results as confirming some of the suspicions which had arisen from earlier studies and had led various researchers to conclude that they were seeing evidence of some environmental factor which was depressing sperm counts.

A basic problem facing those who would use human sperm as an indicator of environmental pollution in the same way that earlier researchers used the health of predatory birds such as falcons or eagles is that we know more about the ecology of such birds than we do about the ecology of the sperm. One reason for this is that the falcon or the eagle is visible to the naked eye and is closely watched throughout its life-cycle by hundreds of thousands, if not millions, of keen bird-watchers and scientific ornithologists. Soaring on thermals or swooping after their prey, these birds capture the imagination and have become powerful romantic symbols. Human sperm, by contrast, are invisible to the naked eye and are far from being a subject for polite conversation.

Another reason why environmentalists have tended to focus on birds rather than sperm is that the reproductive failure of these feathered victims of such chemical compounds as DDT became, ultimately, indisputable. It was no longer simply a question of ornithologists writing learned papers on the unusually thin shells of eggs they had studied in various eyries: anyone who cared to take a walk in the countryside was likely to trip over the evidence, in the form of dead birds, dead foxes and the other biological fallout which followed the widespread, relatively uncontrolled use of the new synthetic insecticides. With sperm, on the other hand, the question of whether sperm counts have actually declined significantly in recent years is still the subject of sometimes bitter controversy.

A landmark study of sperm counts and sperm quality was carried out in 1951 by Dr John MacLeod, Professor of Anatomy, Obstetrics and Gynaecology at Cornell University Medical College in New York. His study, which covered 2,000 fertile and infertile males, confirmed the findings of earlier studies in 1929 and 1938 which suggested that the average sperm count of the fertile male population was above 100 million sperm cells per millilitre of semen, while the infertile population had an average count of ninety million. Dr MacLeod's research was so thorough and so soundly based that it was taken as a standard reference against which other studies were assessed or compared.

Then, in 1973 and 1977, researchers at the University of Iowa and the University of Texas analysed the semen of men about to undergo vasectomy operations – and found that their average sperm counts were dramatically lower than had been reported in those earlier studies. One of these researchers, Dr Raymond Bunge, at the time a physician at the University of Iowa Hospitals, concluded, 'The standards of fertility as determined by semen analysis established by MacLeod in 1950 no longer hold true.' He suggested that 'something has altered the fertile population to depress the semen analysis remarkably. This is obviously speculative, but the overall decrease in the sperm concentration and the semen volumes would tend to incriminate an environmental factor to which the entire population has been exposed.' Bunge, in fact, later extended his speculation to cover the possibility that the growing use of pesticides and herbicides might be one of the underlying causes of the trend.

But there were still scientists who reported that their data did not support the notion that there was a long-term downward trend in sperm counts, including MacLeod himself. He noted in 1979, some twenty-eight years after that landmark study was published, that the data from his laboratory in New York showed no clear trend over the previous three decades. Since at the time these data were unique in being the largest set available from a single laboratory and in covering such a long time span, MacLeod's conclusions were seen as reassuring by many of those working in the field. But there were those who felt that there were still some grounds for concern: MacLeod's data, for example, only covered men involved in infertile matings and no one had yet offered a wholly convincing explanation of the low counts reported by other researchers. However, when a researcher at the Galton Laboratory, University College London, tracked down all the published data he could find on semen samples taken from unselected fertile (or presumably fertile) men, it became clear that there *had* been a significant decline in the sperm counts from those *reported* in the 1930s, 1940s and 1950s to those *reported* in the 1960s and 1970s. The researcher, W. H. James, then reviewed some of the possible explanations for this observed trend.

The first possible explanation was sperm counting errors, various reports suggesting that different technicians could come up with different sperm counts from the same semen samples. To add to the problem, such measurement errors, which might lead to counts being out by as much as ten million sperm per millilitre of semen, may prove to be dwarfed by natural biological variation in sperm counts. Indeed, it has been found that sperm counts are influenced by sexual activity: for every consecutive day of sexual abstinence, a man's sperm count may increase by as much as thirteen million sperm cells.

Given that many of the samples were taken from men about to undergo vasectomy operations another possible influence on the more recent counts is the psychological state of the donor. Stress and other factors, it has been argued, could affect such counts, although some of the recent samples which have shown low counts have been taken from men at institutions other than vasectomy clinics. Some of these, like prisons, have produced remarkably high sperm counts, which have been attributed to a lack of stress and to enforced abstinence, a finding which triggered a different train of thought.

The fact that abstinence can increase sperm counts, and the fact that there is some evidence that married couples, at least in the United States, were engaging somewhat more frequently in inter-course during the period 1965–70, together suggested the possi-bility that the latest semen samples had been taken after shorter periods of sexual abstinence, leading to the reported low sperm counts. But this explanation seems unlikely to be the only one. Roughly speaking, the decline in sperm counts seems to have involved a drop from reported counts of about 100 million per millilitre of semen (prior to 1960) to about 60 million in more recent years. This difference of about 40 million is itself roughly equivalent to the effect of three days' abstinence. Since men in the 1940s were apparently reporting intercourse on average once or twice a week, three days' less abstinence on the part of today's males would suggest something like a doubling of the sexual activity rate over the intervening years – a conclusion which is not borne out by the relevant studies.

In short, the evidence suggested that there had been a real decline in sperm counts, even when such factors were taken into account. But what did this mean for male fertility? Babies were still being born in their millions, and the medical profession was not yet reporting that it was being overwhelmed by a flood-tide of male infertility – so how could sperm quality be assessed?

One possible technique, which has been used extensively in testing the fertility of men whose mothers had been treated with the controversial synthetic oestrogen, diethylstilbestrol (DES), is the 'sperm penetration assay'. Developed by researchers at the University of Hawaii, this assay technique uses denuded hamster eggs as targets for human sperm, to test the sperm's fertilizing capacity. Stripped of their outer membrane, the hamster eggs are incubated in the laboratory and, after exposure to sperm, are examined microscopically for evidence of swelling or decondensing sperm heads in the egg cytoplasm – which would indicate sperm penetration. Those using the assay stress that you do not end up with a human–hamster hybrid, or 'humster'; but the sperm of infertile men, it turns out, rarely penetrate the denuded hamster eggs.

When a research group at the University of Washington looked at the sperm of men whose mothers had been treated with DES, it found that, although low sperm counts were something of a rarity, their sperm often showed a low mobility. Using the sperm penetration assay, it was found that fourteen out of seventeen DES-exposed men tested had an abnormal fertilizing capacity, compared to only one out of eleven semen samples taken from a control group of men who were not exposed to DES. In another control group, made up of men whose wives were actually pregnant at the time of the study, every sperm specimen achieved penetration. A more detailed account of the effect of DES on the outcome of human reproduction can be found in Chapter 4 (p. 110).

There are those who argue that such tests are unreliable or that, even if they are reliably signalling some real problem in the test sperm, we do not yet know enough to interpret those signals with any degree of confidence. One critic, a former University of Washington Associate Professor of Urology, has been quoted as saying that 'nobody knows what the test means'. Dr Mark Kiviat also asserted: 'It's hocus pocus. These cats at the University of Hawaii found that infertile men's sperm had difficulty penetrating denuded hamster eggs. The question is what it means. It's obvious that there are multiple factors involved in male fertility. They're using a test the significance of which is not certain.'

But at least scientists are now seriously looking for tests which will accurately signal problems in sperm samples. The impact of twentieth-century living on human sperm quality remains something of a dark continent, with some recent findings emerging almost by accident – just as Columbus found America while looking for an alternative route to India. For example, the systematic investigation of the effects of paternal drug ingestion on reproductive outcome stemmed from unplanned observations made in the course of experiments designed to identify such effects in female rats exposed to narcotic analgesics. Male rats, caged for mating with female rats receiving methadone or morphine in their drinking water, were themselves exposed to one of the two narcotics. It was discovered that the litters these males later sired with drug-free females showed much higher pre-weaning mortality rates.

When Dr Justin Joffe, Professor of Psychology at the University of Vermont, reviewed the scientific literature on the adverse effects of drugs and chemicals on the progeny of male mammals exposed prior to mating, he quickly found evidence of such effects in five species exposed to seven different chemical agents. The effects of two of these, lead and ethanol, had been known for over fifty years, while those of others (including caffeine and thalidomide) have only been discovered fairly recently.

Despite variations in the species of laboratory animal used, in the chemical agents administered, in the dose and in its timing, three main effects were found in study after study: decreased litter size, decreased birth weights for those animals actually born, and an increased mortality rate for the newborn animals. Different species respond in markedly different ways to any given pollutant or other chemical challenge, which makes it very difficult to draw conclusions about any human response from such animal tests. As Dr Joffe concluded however, 'the demonstration of effects on progeny of paternally-ingested drugs and chemicals in animal experiments carried out under well controlled laboratory conditions establishes the reality of the phenomenon. It permits one to view the less systematic clinical data on humans with less suspicion or, at least, without the conviction that data relating to paternal drug ingestion to sequelae in progeny necessarily have to be explained in a manner that avoids attributing a causal role to paternal drug ingestion.' In other words, if male rats, guinea pigs, rabbits or hamsters exposed to drugs or chemicals are siring smaller and less healthy litters, then the chances are that something of the same may be found in the species which produced those drugs or chemicals in the first place.

Anyone trying to pin particular foetal or child health problems on paternal exposure to particular chemical agents is still likely to find the work tough going at times. In the case of drugs, there is an element of self-selection on the part of those who take them or are treated with them, while the contribution of environmental pollution can be particularly hard to track down. We are told, for example that the lead poisoning of women in the Roman Empire, a process which was unwittingly accelerated by the relaxation of rules forbidding wives from drinking wine – often drunk from lead vessels – was partly responsible for depressing the reproductive capacity of the ruling classes. Falling fertility rates do appear to have been a problem, although it is impossible to be precise about the range of effects experienced. As we shall see later, however, studies of nineteenth- and twentieth-century lead workers and their families have shown smaller-than-normal family sizes, an increased rate of miscarriages among female lead workers and among wives of male lead workers, and an increased mortality rate among the young children of lead workers.

The evidence of increased spontaneous abortion rates and other reproductive problems found among the wives of male anaesthetists is discussed in Chapter 3. Significantly, the rates of congenital abnormalities also show an increase in the children of the wives of three groups of men working in operating theatres: physicians, nurses and operating room technicians.

Two much more commonly used substances also illustrate the nature of the problem, as well as some of the hurdles to be surmounted before real-world causes of human ill-health can be pinpointed accurately. Take the caffeine which most of us drink daily in coffee. Some researchers suspect that such agents as alcohol, caffeine and tobacco derivatives may interact in the human body, complicating the detective work needed to identify culprits in long-term health studies. However, by using predominantly Mormon populations, whose consumption of alcohol, coffee and tobacco is low, some American doctors have produced evidence indicating an unusually high rate of reproductive failure (including spontaneous abortions, stillbirths and premature births) when the father's caffeine consumption was high.

As for smoking, the finding that maternal smoking increased the risk of premature or low-weight babies has been repeatedly confirmed, but it is increasingly being recognized that the father's smoking habits have to be taken into consideration too. It has been shown, for example, that if the father is a smoker while the mother is not, there is no significant increase in the number of low-birth-weight babies born. If, on the other hand, the mother is a smoker and the father smokes too, then there may be a statistically significant increase in low-birth-weight babies among white Americans – but not, apparently, among black Americans.

To complicate matters further, a greater proportion of low-birth-weight babies are likely to die if their fathers smoke than if they do not. Indeed, the highest rates of mortality among low-birth-weight infants were found in the offspring of non-smoking mothers fathered by men who smoke. But, as the researchers pointed out at the time, smokers and non-smokers differ in so many other respects, including their consumption of alcohol and coffee, that it is almost impossible at the moment to point a finger at any single agent as *the* problem.

For one thing, we are still far from sure how any such effects are being transmitted to the newly fertilized human egg. One obvious route would be damage to the sperm itself, which could take such forms as reduced ribosomal activity. Ribosomes, which are found in the cytoplasm of cells, appear to be the site of protein synthesis – so that reduced ribosomal activity can result in impaired protein synthesis. This possibility is suggested by the fact that the amount of ribonucleic acid (RNA) found in the testes of rats exposed to lead was significantly lower than in the testes of lead-free rats.

Another possibility is that chromosomal damage is occurring, perhaps resulting in a lethal mutation. But a contradictory indication is the finding that rodents exposed to chemicals such as ethanol are more likely to show reproductive defects if subjected to a single dose or short-term exposure than they are if subjected to long-term exposure. There can be no doubt, as we shall see, that some chemicals can cause chromosomal damage, but it is still far from clear that paternal exposure is significant in this respect.

A second route would involve the transmission to the fertilized egg of drugs, or of drug or chemical metabolites (break-down products), in the semen itself. In experiments with rabbits, for example, thalidomide and its metabolites were found to be present in appreciable amounts in the semen of the experimental animals. In humans, methadone has been found in the semen of patients at one American clinic. The presence of such drugs in semen suggests a number of ways in which paternally ingested drugs or chemicals might influence the health of any offspring. They might affect sperm motility, for example, which would account for any decline in paternal fertility and perhaps also for decreased litter sizes in experimental animals. Such effects are found in human patients undergoing anticonvulsant therapy and among heroin users.

Another possibility is that drugs and chemicals in the semen might have some effect on the uterus, either directly or by means of uterine absorption, possibly affecting the timing of blastocyst implantation (see Figure 4.1, p. 93), the distribution of implantation sites or the development of the placenta. Cases which have been reported of women developing an allergic reaction to their partners' sperm also suggest that semen itself in some instances, and in others possibly contaminants in the semen, may be altering the uterine environment in ways which may be detrimental to the developing embryo.

A third route could involve alterations in the volume or chemical make-up of the semen, with morphine among the drugs which have been shown to reduce the rate of secretions from rat seminal vesicles and methadone ingestion shown to be related to a reduction of over 50 per cent in the volume of semen produced by man. Such changes could clearly have a detrimental effect on sperm transport, and thereby on fertilization, while any chemical which, say, affected the levels of such natural components of semen as prostaglandin would also be of interest, since prostaglandins are thought to be involved in sperm transport and fertilization.

Two chemical compounds which have been found to have a profound impact on the fertility of men exposed to them are dibromochloropropane (DBCP), used as a soil fumigant and nematocide, and chlordecone (better known as Kepone), the pesticide which, for a time, ranked as the most publicized toxin – ceding place only to that toxin of toxins, dioxin.

Kepone (or decachlorooctahydro-1,3,4-metheno-2H-cyclobuta-(c,d)pentalen-2-one, to give it its full chemical name) was first registered by Allied Chemical Company in 1952 for the control of ants and cockroaches. It was largely exported to Central and South America, via Germany, for use against the banana root borer. In Europe, Kepone has mainly been used against potato beetles and had been manufactured for years without any known harmful effects on the workers producing it.

As so often happens, however, once a problem emerges, you can pinpoint evidence which emerged a good deal earlier and signalled danger. Allied Chemical itself never seems to have hit the problems which surfaced when Life Science Products Company entered the picture in 1973, although experiments carried out on behalf of Allied Chemical between 1958 and 1961 had shown that Kepone could kill with chronic exposure (which was perhaps not particularly surprising) and that increasing doses led to increasing numbers of test animals showing testicular atrophy.

Similar effects showed up in other test animals such as the rabbit, and the evidence from mammals strongly suggested that, over a long period of time, adverse effects on the testes could be triggered at doses as low as 10 parts per million of Kepone in the animals' diet, a dose which was well below that required for outright symptoms of toxicity. There was also some evidence that the condition was reversible if the animals were withdrawn from exposure to the pesticide, although experiments on birds such as pheasants showed that Kepone not only inhibited their reproduction but also produced irreversible damage to the testicles of the males. One part per million of Kepone was found to have a marked effect on pheasant reproduction; 25 ppm put an almost total brake on reproduction; and at doses of 50 ppm male pheasants developed female plumage and abnormal testes and showed misshapen spermatozoa.

Kepone, like other organochlorine compounds with a high fat solubility, has been found to concentrate in human breast milk. Significant levels appeared in the breast milk of women who had been in an area sprayed with Mirex, a similar cyclodiene insecticide (also used for the control of fire ants and manufactured as a fire retardant under the name dechlorane). Mirex's breakdown products include Kepone.

The real problems began when, in March 1973, Allied decided to give a tolling contract (involving licensing another company to manufacture a product, in this case Kepone) to Life Science Products, which had recently been established by two of Allied's ex-employees. The plant where the pesticide had been manufactured was needed by Allied's plastics division, and there was no reason to expect any particular problems with what was a routine decision: Kepone had already been toll manufactured by Hooker Chemical and by Nease Chemical.

The two ex-Allied men were William P. Moore, who had been director of research at Allied's agricultural division for some years, and Virgil A. Hundtofte, who had been an Allied plant manager in Hopewell, Virginia, which was destined to become the epicentre of the Kepone affair. Both had experience of manufacturing Kepone. Just in case Moore and Hundtofte had forgotten any details, Allied supplied Life Science Products with a detailed manual on Kepone manufacture, a manual which stressed the need for such protective measures as respirators and gloves for those working in a Kepone production plant, as well as a shower before workers left the plant for home. But if Moore and Hundtofte ever read the manual, it failed to show in their day-to-day running of the Life Science Products operation.

As it later transpired, workers often ate lunch in the factory itself, munching their sandwiches while surrounded by Kepone dust. When Dr Robert S. Jackson, the State of Virginia's chief epidemiologist, investigated one case of what had become familiarly known as the 'Kepone shakes', he was appalled to find Kepone dust lying several centimetres deep in some places as he walked around the plant. And, he found, the Life Science Products workers had been ignoring even the most elementary safety precautions.

By the summer of 1975, some sixteen months after Life Science Products first started toll manufacture of Kepone, a number of workers were suffering from severe headaches and tremors. Some were later found to be sterile. And monitoring studies showed that not only did some of the workers' wives and children have traces of Kepone in their blood, but the entire area around the plant had become heavily contaminated. The Hopewell sewage treatment plant had been put out of action and research carried out at the Environmental Protection Agency's laboratory at Research Triangle park showed that the James tidal river and estuary was also badly polluted. EPA scientists found concentrations of Kepone as high as 2.1 milligrams per gram in finned fish caught in the river and 0.48 milligrams per gram in oysters.

Governor Mills Godwin promptly closed the entire James river and its tributaries for the harvest of finned fish and shellfish, to protect public health. An indication of the gravity of the problem is that the Governor went for closure even though the private oyster industry in Virginia was almost entirely dependent on seed oysters taken from the lower James river. These are harvested and sold to watermen from other areas of Chesapeake Bay. After replanting, the oysters grow to market size over about three years. With some 70 per cent of the Virginia private oyster industry dependent on the lower James river, the Governor knew he had problems: if the 1976 seed harvest was interrupted, there would be no 1979 oyster harvest.

Research was then carried out in short order at the Virginia Institute of Marine Sciences, Gloucester Point, to see whether the seed oysters could be purged of Kepone contamination in time to avoid this impending commercial calamity. Experiments showed that with summer temperatures, oysters could purge themselves of the contamination after two weeks in clean water, so the harvest was allowed to go ahead. But the harvesting of other river and marine species was controlled or banned for years afterwards. As the Kepone gradually sank into the river's mud, the controls were relaxed, so that by 1983 recreational and some commercial fishing were again permitted. Rex Crawford, who worked for the Virginia Commission of Game and Inland Fisheries, was then quoted as saying he had no doubts about eating fish caught in the James, although he qualified his statement by saying, 'But then again, I smoke.'

Meanwhile, back at the Hopewell plant, the Virginia State Health Department was finding it rather harder than it had expected to track down the workers who might have been exposed to Kepone over those critical sixteen months prior to shut-down. The turnover of staff had been so high, not least because of the appalling conditions in the plant, that the workforce had been effectively replaced five times. Eventually, the Department identified thirty-three current employees and 115 former employees, and tracked down all but fifteen of these for medical check-up. In addition, some 270 family members, thirty-nine Allied employees and 214 people selected from the neighbourhood were investigated.

The three symptoms reported most frequently by those studied were a sense of nervousness, tremors (particularly in the hands, but sometimes affecting the entire body), and difficulties in focusing the eyes, a condition which sometimes erupted into rapid, erratic eye movements. As far as reproductive toxicology went, the investigators found low sperm counts and an unusual proportion of abnormal and non-motile sperm in the samples taken from present and past workers.

As far as the general community was concerned, a small number of people turned out to have Kepone traces in their blood, although none showed clinical symptoms of Kepone poisoning. Two of the workers' wives, however, showed indisputable tremors and other family members had Kepone in their blood. Because Kepone is highly soluble in fat, it can take a very long time to flush out of the body, being eliminated mainly in the bile and faeces. Treatment with cholestyramine was found to accelerate the excretion rate and, ultimately, most of those whose sperm counts had been affected by Kepone were found to have recovered.

Paradoxically, Allied had prided itself on being an environmentally responsible company. Indeed, its top managers were unaware that they were sitting on such a time-bomb. 'This has been the most shocking experience of my business career,' said John T. Connor, the company's chairman. In the event, Allied's handling of the problem, once it had surfaced, was little short of exemplary. For example, when it emerged that Life Science Products was on the verge of bankruptcy, Connor ensured that Allied assumed responsibility for cleaning up the Hopewell plant. Because the plant was so heavily contaminated, normal decontamination procedures were considered to be insufficient, and Allied spent $394,000 on dismantling and dumping the dismembered factory and machinery in a sealed pit at the Hopewell waste disposal site. So superheated was the political atmosphere that even when Allied had treated water from the plant such that, in the words of one company official, it was 'purer than most drinking water', no one was prepared to permit its disposal. Eventually, however, the Environmental Protection Agency relented, and the water was sprayed on some company land in the Hopewell area.

Clearly, Connor should have been able to close this highly unfortunate chapter in Allied's history at this stage, and he certainly responded by pulling environmental concerns very much higher up the list of management priorities. But he found he was dealing with a chain reaction of events. A veritable swarm of state and federal investigators descended on the Hopewell plant in the wake of the first cases of Kepone poisoning, going through the company's records with the proverbial fine-toothed comb. And Connor soon found himself in an even worse position.

Leafing through old files, an investigator from the Environmental Protection Agency found an error in a form filled by Allied in 1971 which, in effect, meant that the company had been discharging Kepone and two polymers into the James river without a permit. Probing deeper, it was found that the plant's manager at the time had been none other than Virgil Hundtofte, later a co-founder of Life Science Products. Hundtofte claimed that he had been confused by the form, drawn up by the Corps of Engineers. Anyone who has seen some of the forms which industrialists now have to complete might sympathize, but Hundtofte's case fell apart when new evidence emerged.

A memorandum was discovered which, in American legal parlance, turned out to be the 'smoking gun'. This made it quite clear that Hundtofte had realized that the form required that he identify the three pollutants, but he apparently feared that if the Environmental Protection Agency found out that they were being discharged, Allied would be forced to suspend production and to install pollution control plant costing perhaps $700,000. When one considers that Kepone was a fairly minor product for Allied, never producing a net profit of more than $600,000 a year, the logic becomes clear. Hundtofte hoped that, at best, a problem ignored might be a problem solved or, at worst, time might be bought so that the plant could later hook into a planned regional water-treatment facility, avoiding the suspension of production and the cost of new pollution control plant.

And then it became known that the National Cancer Institute was on the verge of publishing a study suggesting that Kepone could cause cancer. Published early in 1976, the study showed that a significant proportion of test mice and rats fed Kepone developed liver cancer. Despite the difficulties involved in drawing conclusions from animal tests about any effects in humans, and despite the fact that DDT, which is chemically similar to Kepone, had not produced a single indisputable human cancer after decades of animal tests suggesting that it was a carcinogen, the National Cancer Institute's finding was another nail in Allied's legal coffin.

Faced with a bankrupt Life Science Products, the company's workers decided to sue Allied for a total of $186.3 million; some 400 fishermen, oystermen and others affected by the ban on fishing in the James river sued for $24 million; a 'class action' for an astonishing $8.5 billion was filed on behalf of 10,000 fishermen and those whose business depended on the health of the fishing industry; a group of stockholders filed suit against Allied's board of directors, claiming that it had failed to meet its responsibilities in the Kepone affair; and the Justice Department's proceeding against Allied imposed the maximum penalty – presenting a total bill of $13.2 million, compared with a previous high of $1 million levied against Reserve Mining Company for dumping taconite tailings into Lake Superior.

By a good deal of legal juggling, Allied managed to settle most of these actions at very much lower levels, so that its total bill was more like $25 million on the legal front. But the blow to the company's public prestige was enormous. In his final ruling for the Justice Department, Judge Robert R. Mehrige, Jr, well known for taking a stand on such issues, accepted that Allied was typically a 'good corporate citizen' but felt that a heavy fine was needed to deter others. 'I hope after this sentence that every corporate official, every corporate employee, that has any reason to think pollution is going on,' he said, 'will think: "If I don't do something about it now, I am apt to be out of a job tomorrow".'

Industrial apologists might say, with some justification, that Allied was unfairly treated, particularly in the light of its highly responsible conduct once the problem came to light. They might also point to the fact that those exposed to Kepone ultimately recovered. But the fact remains that large numbers of people were exposed to a totally unacceptable degree of risk from a chemical whose dangers should have been suspected from the available animal test results. And, in some respects, Allied was lucky. It could have been dealing with a compound like dibromochloropropane (DBCP). Men exposed to DBCP during manufacturing or field spraying operations were found to have depressed sperm counts and testicular damage, damage which in the most severely affected cases proved irreversible.

It is a modern paradox that while companies like Allied are being forced to devote ever increasing efforts to the protection of human sperm, other groups around the world are devoting ever increasing efforts to research on chemical means for shutting off sperm production. At the Pasteur Institute in Paris, for example, French scientists have been working on what has been dubbed 'immunological castration', involving the development of a vaccine which could be used instead of surgical castration in farm and domestic animals. Similar work is proceeding in relation to human sperm, for if there is one thing we undoubtedly have too much of, it is human sperm. In contrast to the situation prevailing in the bloodstock industry, where a stallion such as the kidnapped Shergar can earn £70,000 for each foal sired, there is no market for human sperm – and it is therefore impossible to place a value on partial or total sterility.

Of course, in this brave new world of ours, things are changing.

The Xytex Corporation, for example, which is based in Augusta, Georgia, is one of a new breed of industrial concerns which is aiming to establish a thriving market in human sperm: it sends out frozen sperm by mail order to doctors carrying out artificial insemination, supplying catalogues listing donors with details of their ethnic origin, height, weight, hair and eye colour, skin colour and blood group. The service, apparently, costs 'well under $100' and donors are paid between $20 and $40 per sample.

In spite of this, and regardless of whether we are looking for male birth control vaccines or drugs and of whether or not we can attach a value to particular samples of semen, the fact is that some industrial activities are imposing unwanted sterility on workers – and the discovered problems are, in the way of things, likely to be the tip of a somewhat larger iceberg.

If one looks at these problems objectively, it is quite clear that depressed sperm counts and damaged testicles, despite the psychological impact on those whose reproductive capacity is affected, are very much second or third division problems when compared with the dreadful damage some chemicals and drugs can wreak on the human embryo and foetus. Yet there are dangers in trying to attach priority rankings to human reproductive problems in this way. Ultimately, just as when we are dealing with a natural ecosystem, we are working with a highly complex and inter-related system whose parts are interdependent in ways we may not even guess at. While the cynic might shrug off the evidence of the damage we are doing in terms of falling sperm counts on the basis that this is Nature's way of dealing with the population problem, we should be wrong to do so. Whether we work in factories, live alongside them or use their products, we have an unshakeable right to do so without having our health damaged in the process.

And there is also the question of sperm *quality*. While environmental protection and industrial health and safety control agencies may give male sterility a relatively low priority in relation to the problems we are about to consider, there is growing evidence that human sperm can provide a direct route into the womb for many of our most dangerous pollutants. The sperm may yet prove to be the Trojan Horse of reproductive toxicology.

CHAPTER THREE

UNBORN
CANARIES

Maybe the little yellow bird simply stopped singing, maybe it slumped from its perch to the floor of its cage. Either way, it was enough to alert the miners who had carried the canary to the coal-face that, unseen, unsensed, toxic or inflammable gases were building up around them. Today's miner is more likely to rely on an electronic canary, perhaps based on infra-red spectroscopy. But in communities and workplaces around the planet another tiny creature, crouched in its darkened cage, is signalling that all is far from well with the world. The creature is the human foetus, the cage its mother's womb.

Rachel Carson saw it coming. Commenting on the evidence that the suckling infant often takes in toxic chemicals with its mother's milk, she stressed that 'it is by no means his first exposure'. Indeed, she continued: 'There is good reason to believe this begins while he is still in the womb. In experimental animals the chlorinated hydrocarbon insecticides freely cross the barrier of the placenta, the traditional protective shield between the embryo and harmful substances in the mother's body.'

The quantities of chemical involved might be readily detectable, or they might seem insignificant but, 'they are not unimportant because children are more susceptible to poisoning than adults. This situation,' she concluded, 'also means that today the average individual almost certainly starts life with the first deposit of the growing load of chemicals his body will be required to carry henceforth.'

In writing *Silent Spring* Rachel Carson was concerned to show that animal or human fat cells can act as 'biological magnifiers', so that an intake of o.1 parts per million of DDT in the diet, say, could result in the storage of 10 to 15 parts per million in the body's fat cells – representing a hundred-fold amplification, or even worse. In many respects the book, first published in 1962, is astonishingly up to date, but some areas of environmental and medicinal science have developed considerably in the intervening years and none more so than reproductive toxicology.

Yet when a research team from the pharmacology department at Guy's Hospital Medical School, London, was asked by the UK Health and Safety Executive to review the available evidence on the reproductive toxicity of some fifty widely used industrial chemicals, the team concluded that there were still yawning information gaps to be filled. Although research on the reproductive toxicity of industrial chemicals is now one of the fastest-growing areas of concern in toxicology, Susan Barlow and Frank Sullivan reported, 'This is not yet matched by any substantial body of reliable evidence that would permit some assessment of the extent of the potential problem.'

Despite these information gaps, however, the team stressed, 'It is clear, from both experiments in animals and epidemiological studies in humans, that industrial chemicals do have the potential to cause reproductive toxicity.' And, as will become clear below, the effects which reproductive toxicologists are now concerned with turn up not only in the womb but, in one direction, before conception even takes place and, in the other, beyond birth, as the surviving children continue to develop.

When the American Cyanamid Corporation found itself at the centre of an acrimonious and highly publicized controversy in 1979, following the discovery by the media that five women employed at the company's Willow Island plant had opted for sterilization in order to keep their jobs, few people realized that this was simply the latest in a long line of skirmishes within the very substantial sector of industry which uses lead-based raw materials.

William Island grabbed the headlines because it highlighted a wider problem women were encountering in their attempts to gain employment in manufacturing industries. As Ronald Bayer of the Hastings Center put it, Willow Island became 'a symbol of a new and very bitter phase in the struggle between workers and corporation over the question of occupational health and safety. But in this case a second feature made the confrontation all the more acrimonious. Women who, as a result of civil rights legislation and court action, had begun to break the male monopoly over relatively high-paying blue-collar jobs were now being threatened with dismissals, demotions, or barriers to employment in the name of fetal health.'

This time, however, they were to be restricted because they bore a special responsibility to future generations – a responsibility which might be prejudiced if mothers or potential mothers were exposed to workplace chemicals suspected of causing birth defects or mutations. Among the companies which decided to exclude women from certain high-risk jobs were Allied Chemical, Du Pont, General Motors, Gulf Oil, Monsanto, Olin, Sun Oil and Union Carbide. Estimates of the numbers of jobs closed to women because of the resulting policies ranged upwards from a 'conservative' 100,000. Indeed, the US Equal Employment Opportunity Commission and the Office of Federal Contract Compliance Programs concluded that if all suspect chemicals were seriously considered (including benzene, carbon monoxide, carbon tetrachloride, lead and vinyl chloride), as many as twenty million jobs could be involved in the United States alone.

In an argument which closely echoes that used by many of the companies and corporations now using (or planning to use) some of the new genetic screening techniques, Dow Chemical's director of health and environmental services explained that 'the difficulty and cost of implementing good industrial hygiene shouldn't be used as a blanket excuse to exclude women. But if the cost is going to rise exponentially to reach a certain level for uniquely fetal toxins, it's justified to take them out of the workplace then.'

Some critics took the line that these new exclusionary policies were encouraging women to exchange their reproductive capacity for employment. American Cyanamid might have offered other jobs to the five at Willow Island, they say, but the alternatives involved lower rates of pay. Another line of attack was adopted by those who saw the trend towards exclusionary policies as a serious challenge to the right of all workers to a safe working environment. Whereas these industrial corporations had tried to justify their policies by classifying all fertile women and the foetuses of any pregnant women as 'hypersusceptibles', organizations such as the US Council on Environmental Quality (CEQ) argued that the scientific evidence suggesting that men were less susceptible was totally inadequate.

Far from the evidence suggesting that women and foetuses were the only 'hypersusceptibles', the CEQ argued, there was some evidence that the foetus could be harmed following the exposure to suspect industrial chemicals of the father alone. This line of argument was supported by Eula Bingham, as head of the US Occupational Safety and Health Administration (OSHA), which had insisted, during the Carter administration, that industry should adopt standards which protect even the most vulnerable workers from harm.

'We must stand firm on the principle that if an exposure is sufficiently toxic to produce genetic damage in an unborn child or in a fertile female,' the director of the US National Institute of Occupational Safety and Health (NIOSH) argued, 'then it must be considered to be equally toxic to the fertile male worker and to the unborn child.' As director of NIOSH, he was writing to one of the corporations which had decided to adopt an exclusionary policy – and he concluded that 'there is *a priori* no reason to believe that the genetic material of a male worker is any more resistant to toxic occupational injury than that of the female'. But if one looks back at the history of the lead industry, it is apparent that the emphasis of any efforts to control the impact of lead exposure on the human reproductive cycle has almost invariably been to remove pregnant women from the workplace. The Guy's Hospital Medical School team, which used very rigorous standards in evaluating the credibility of reproductive toxicology research data, found that the 'first systematic reports linking reproductive effects to an industrial chemical were on lead toxicity and were published towards the end of the nineteenth century, culminating at the turn of the century in the banning of women from work in many of the heavy lead-using trades'.

Significantly, abnormally high rates of infertility, spontaneous abortion, stillbirth, macrocephaly (unusually large head or skull), convulsions and early deaths had long been reported among the offspring of people living and working with high lead exposures. And, equally interesting, many of these reports suggested that such exposures could affect the reproductive capacity of both men and women – although it was generally unclear whether the problems reported stemmed from direct exposure of the mothers to lead (either in the workplace or on their husbands' working

clothes), from exposure to environmental lead in the neighbourhood of lead-using industries, or from the exposure of their
husbands to lead. More recently, however, research has shown
that at blood lead levels which are commonly found in high lead-
level working situations, male workers will typically have a lower
sperm count – and the sperm that remain will be more likely
to be misshapen and less mobile than unaffected sperm.

Strangely, though, despite this early evidence of the chemical
disruption of the human reproductive cycle, this whole area went
largely unresearched for many years. The one field in which there
was continuing, if initially sporadic, interest in reproductive effects
was radiation medicine. Research was carried out on people
exposed to intense nuclear fallout after the explosion of atomic
bombs (whether during the Second World War in Japan or later
in atomic tests such as those carried out in the Marshall Islands),
on uranium miners and on workers in the luminizing industry.

Much of the work on radiation focused on fatal cancers, which
are the most important late effect of radiation exposure, but
another important effect is hereditary damage – the probability
(but not severity) of which depends on the radiation dose received.
The damage arises when the human gonads, which produce the
sperm cells in males and the egg cells in females, are irradiated.
Ionizing radiation induces mutations which in most cases are
harmful to such cells.

There is also the risk to children irradiated in the womb, with
the evidence suggesting that such irradiation can lead to a wide
range of developmental problems or to malignant disease in childhood. As with women working in the lead-using industries, fertile
women are typically subject to special restrictions on the doses
they may receive when employed as radiation workers – and
pregnant women are rarely given abdominal X-ray examinations.

Even after the thalidomide disaster, the idea that industrial
chemicals could cause problems for the unborn did not really catch
on. What really began to tip the scales was the evidence of severe
neurological damage reported in newborn babies in the Minamata
and Niigata areas of Japan, with 6 per cent of all births affected by
what became known as Minamata disease. What particularly
struck the medical profession was the irrefutable evidence that the
developing embryo and foetus were unusually sensitive to environmental chemicals – with a number of the affected children being

born to mothers who had themselves shown no obvious symptoms.

As a direct result, and in the wake of later disasters involving exposure to pesticides such as chlordecone or dibromochloropropane, and to such materials as dioxin or vinyl chloride monomer, the remit of reproductive toxicologists was dramatically extended. Increasingly, they were interested not only in chemicals which were known to kill the embryo or foetus, but also in sublethal effects extending across the entire reproductive cycle, from the exposure of the mother or father prior to conception through to defects in the children such as mental retardation or cancers.

Such problematic materials as lead can affect reproduction in two ways: they can build up directly in the reproductive organs of the parents and in the tissue of the developing foetus or, indirectly, they can disrupt some of the physiological processes involved in human reproduction. As far as direct effects are concerned, lead has been shown to accumulate in a number of organs which are vital to reproductive success, including the gonads, hypothalamus and pituitary gland. Lead can cross the placental barrier and, in experimental animals at least, has been found in the mother's milk.

And, as Dr Ellen Silbergeld of the Environmental Defense Fund has pointed out, 'nonspecific toxic effects of lead may also compromise reproduction indirectly. For example, the behavioral toxicity of lead, which alters social interactions and reactivity, may adversely affect sexual receptivity and the complex behavioral patterns involved in mating.' But Dr Silbergeld's observations were based on animal experiments and, as she recognized, it is no easy task to reach conclusions about human sexual behaviour by studying rodent reproduction.

What do we know about the effect of chemicals on the various stages of the human reproductive cycle? Let's take each stage of the development of a child in turn and consider some of the relevant research findings that have emerged in recent years. What follows is clearly not intended to be an encyclopaedic classification of all the effects known to occur, nor is it meant to be a minute-by-minute account of the development of a fertilized egg into a fully-fledged human being. We have seen how some industrial chemicals can affect human sperm counts and sperm motility, and the way in which irradiation can affect the gonads – the ovaries and the testes. These effects can be quantified but some others, while they may be real enough, are harder to pin down.

Consider the sexual urge itself. Reproductive toxicologists distinguish between libido, the desire to engage in sexual intercourse, and potency, the ability to do so. Both libido and potency can be affected in a number of ways. Chemicals or other agents can interfere with hormone secretion, or they may affect the central nervous system. Other toxic effects, or psychological problems following the realization that exposure to a potentially hazardous chemical has taken place, can also affect libido and potency.

There have been reports of workers exposed to tetraethyl lead in petrol complaining of reduced libido and potency, complaints which were backed up with research that showed reduced semen volume and reduced sperm counts, together with significant abnormalities in the sperm themselves. When these men were removed from the source of the organic lead, potency apparently soon returned but, sadly, no one thought to check whether their sperm counts, which remained low for some time, eventually recovered.

A much more detailed study was carried out on a group of six men who complained of loss of libido after exposure to metallic mercury vapour in an industrial accident in which a mercury-containing thermostat broke and more than 10 millilitres of mercury were vaporized in an oven. Of the nine men on the night shift, six were hospitalized, all presenting symptoms typical of acute mercury poisoning including fever, chills and chest pains. Unusually, all six were followed up over a period of years. While their chronic symptoms differed to some degree, they all complained of an increased nervousness, irritability, lack of ambition and, the real point of interest here, a lack of sexual desire.

In this case, unlike that of the men exposed to tetraethyl lead, libido and potency were badly affected – and for very considerable periods of time. In one case, the loss of interest in sex coincided with the onset of a shaking tremor, a clumsy gait, irritability and suspiciousness. The abnormal gait and the tremor persisted for two years after the accident, but then slowly disappeared. After five years, this man's handwriting had returned to normal but, significantly, he never regained an interest in sex.

The second case involved a loss of libido spanning two years, and the third and fourth cases lost their sexual appetite for eight years. The fifth case complained that eighteen months after the accident he was suddenly unable to have an erection, although this problem cleared after a time. The sixth reported initially losing interest, although he was later able to resume a normal, if somewhat limited, sex life.

This cluster of cases, reported by McFarland and Reigel in 1978, was particularly well documented, whereas the loss of libido following manganese poisoning in Chilean miners focused on men who had been pensioned off from a mine some years previously – indeed up to twenty-five years previously. All thirteen of the chronically poisoned miners examined, however, were severely affected by a permanently crippling neurological disease involving disorders in their gait, speech and reflexes. Eight of the men examined in the study reported by Mena et al. complained of sexual impotence, a symptom absent from a control group of healthy miners with the same age range who were studied at the same time. Other studies have found the same effect, with one study reporting that 80 per cent of those poisoned suffered from at least temporary impotence. One possible mechanism which has been suggested is the depression of testosterone secretion in those affected.

Turning to a number of chemicals which are used in synthetic materials, similar effects have been observed in a group of firemen exposed to toluene di-isocyanate while fighting a fire in a factory where polyurethane foam (for which TDI is a raw material) was manufactured. The leakage of TDI was massive, involving a total of 4,500 litres, and the men were in direct contact with the chemical following the soaking of their clothing and equipment. Among the effects reported by those involved were irritability, headaches, poor memory, gastro-enteritis, acute euphoria and even loss of consciousness. Two men complained of impotence lasting for two weeks, although with some of the other symptoms reported this is perhaps not surprising.

Of eighteen firemen examined four years after the fire, thirteen were found to be still clinically affected, experiencing difficulty in concentrating, bouts of depression and irritability. When they were tested for long-term memory, this also showed signs of impairment.

Another material which has been shown to cause loss of libido in exposed workers is vinyl chloride, used in organic syntheses in the plastics industry, in the production of vinyl chloride resins and of methyl chloroform, and as a component in propellants. A number of studies have shown that men exposed to vinyl chloride monomer were liable to suffer a loss of libido. Here again, this loss may have been a result of other symptoms, which included fatigue, aches in the muscles and bones, cold hands and feet, and a loss of grip.

These and other cases suggest that a range of widely used industrial chemicals can depress both libido and potency, although these effects may be difficult to disentangle from a welter of other symptoms. An equally difficult field to assess is the impact of such chemicals on menstruation, with women reporting a fairly wide range of experiences even under normal circumstances.

While investigators have found it harder to assess the impact of exposure to chemicals on women's libido than to assess the impact in men, menstruation is at least a physical cycle whose disruption can be evaluated statistically across a group of women exposed to a particular environmental threat. Disturbances in menstruation, often following disruptions of the hormone release patterns in the hypothalamus, pituitary gland or ovaries, have been observed in rodents, primates and humans, with current suspicions centering on a fairly large group of chemicals. These include aniline, benzene, chloroprene (also implicated in loss of libido and potency), formaldehyde, inorganic mercury, polychlorinated biphenyls, styrene and toluene.

To show that reproductive toxicology problems are no respecters of political frontiers, we shall start with some menstrual disturbances reported in the USSR – where such problems are seen as one indicator of a chemical's potential reproductive toxicity.

The aniline dye industry in the western Urals has been the subject of at least one major study in this field, with examinations carried out on over 1,200 women, followed by interviews. This represented nearly 85 per cent of the women employed in the main and auxiliary workshops of this section of the industry, with just over 80 per cent of the women sampled working in the facilities producing organic dyes, intermediates, and aniline and its derivatives. A control group of women who worked in administrative departments, crèches and playgrounds, who had probably not been exposed to the chemicals used in the production plants, was also involved in the study.

When the study data were analysed, it emerged that there were five main causes for sick leave among the women: diseases of the respiratory, digestive, cardiovascular and skeletomuscular systems and of the urogenitary organs. Dietary factors, which were a major focus of the study, emerged as highly important in determining the frequency of menstrual disturbances, abortions and inflammatory disease of the sex organs. But, significantly, the highest incidences of gynaecological disease was found among women working on the production of organic dyes and intermediates, or employed as machine operators, packers, chemical equipment repairers and laboratory workers.

The most frequent disorder reported was the disturbance of menstrual and ovarian cycles, which occurred in nearly half of the women working in organic chemical production compared with the overall factory incidence of 26 per cent – and a mere 3 per cent among the control group.

Similar problems also emerged among workers exposed to urea-formaldehyde resins in the First Moscow Print works and in the Moscow Three Mountain Fabric cotton combine. The study looked at three groups of women: 130 shop trim finishers, exposed to high environmental levels of formaldehyde released from the resins; 316 warehouse inspectors, exposed to lower levels; and 200 women employed as industrial sales staff, who were not exposed and were examined as controls. Menstrual disorders were found in nearly half (47.5 per cent) of the exposed women, compared to just over a sixth (18.6 per cent) of the controls – the most common problem being dysmenorrhea, involving pains in the abdomen and lower back during periods. The incidence of inflammatory disease of the genital tract was also significantly higher among the finishers, a problem which appeared to be associated with a higher rate of infertility.

Benzene and chloroprene have also been found to contribute to such disorders. Indeed, benzene was once used for a short time as a drug in the treatment of leukaemia, being taken in the form of gelatin-coated capsules. The patients typically died of benzene poisoning before succumbing to the final stages of leukaemia, and the deaths were often associated with menorrhagia – excessive bleeding during periods. As for chloroprene, used in the manufacture of synthetic rubber, a study in the United States found that nearly half of the sixty-five women working in one neoprene rubber glove factory had menstrual disorders, compared to 10 per cent in a control group.

Inorganic mercury is another suspect, with disorders showing up in women working in dentistry, mercury rectifier stations and in the manufacture of fluorescent lamps. A strange finding among the workers producing fluorescent lamps, however, was that the abnormalities seemed to disappear after five years of employment in the factory. The researchers had no idea why this was happening, although they suggested that it might either be because the women were adapting or because women newly employed in the plant had the greatest exposure.

Other materials which are suspected of causing menstrual disorders may rarely be found in isolation, introducing problems of sorting out just which chemical is causing what effect. For example, in the USSR research carried out on toluene was initially reported as showing a higher incidence of menstrual disorders among women working in a plant producing enamel-coated wires – and exposed to synthetic di-electric varnishes. These effects were later attributed to 'the combined effect of various solvents (toluene, xylene, white spirit, and others) and sometimes coupled with other substances' – suggesting that the women involved were exposed to a fair number of chemicals in addition to toluene.

One interesting aspect of human reproduction, and it is true of mammals in general, is that all the eggs that will ever be ovulated are already present at birth, being stored in a form of suspended animation in the ovaries. Fluctuating hormone levels then trigger the release of one or more eggs to begin the cycle of ovulation. Research carried out in the anatomy department of Cambridge University, however, suggests that these stored eggs may be vulnerable even to such a common chemical as alcohol, which appears to interfere with the segregation of chromosomes during egg maturation. The resulting embryos are called aneuploid, because they have an abnormal number of chromosomes.

Given that clinical observations of human spontaneous abortions suggest that between 25 and 30 per cent of all such abortions result from the fact that the embryo is aneuploid, the finding inevitably stirred concern – and it has been suggested that an even greater number of fertilized eggs may be affected, but die soon after implantation on the uterus wall, making this aspect of the problem hard to detect. This research used experimental mice (making its conclusions subject to the various uncertainties outlined in Chapter 7), but the levels of alcohol involved in the experiments, when scaled up to the human equivalents, were only about twice as great as the legal limit for drinking and driving in Britain.

If the human egg passes through the obstacle course described above and meets a sperm which has survived the obstacle course described in the previous chapter, it is by no means home and dry. The next set of challenges come during fertilization and implantation, with the overwhelming majority of abnormal sperm failing to achieve fertilization and the majority of abnormal fertilized eggs failing to achieve sustained implantation.

A chemical may disrupt implantation directly, by affecting the success of fertilization, or indirectly by disrupting a woman's hormonal output and balance. Ovulation may not occur, for example, if there is any interference with the cyclical release from the pituitary of the 'gonadotrophic' hormones, luteinizing hormone and follicle stimulating hormone – which depends on instructions from the hypothalamus and feedback from ovarian hormones. In the same way, implantation is critically dependent on the secretion of ovarian hormones, which prepare the lining of the uterus for the arrival of the blastocyst and which can be disrupted by external agents even if fertilization has been achieved.

If the blastocyst is to implant itself successfully (see Figures 4.1–4.3, p. 93), it must also have an adequate supply through the mother's blood of oxygen and nutrients. Any reduction in the supply of blood or oxygen may either prevent implantation taking place at all or, if it takes place, result in early spontaneous abortion. One threat to the blastocyst, according to research carried out at Wayne State University in Michigan, is smoking. Cigarette smoking is known to increase the incidence of abortion, developmental abnormalities and small-for-term babies, and it is now thought that nicotine can affect the uterine environment even before the blastocyst implants itself, making it less likely that it will be able to do so. Other chemicals in fairly common usage, or to which pregnant mothers are exposed, are proving to have the same effect.

There has been a good deal of controversy, for instance, about the suggestion that anaesthetics used in the operating theatre have increased the rate of spontaneous abortions among female anaesthetists and resulted in a higher rate of congenital abnormalities in the surviving foetuses. In one controlled study in Britain, the abortion rate among anaesthetists (18.2 per cent) was significantly higher than that for non-anaesthetists (14.7 per cent), while the frequency of unplanned, involuntary infertility (12 per cent) was twice that found in control groups (6 per cent). A later study by the same team failed to find evidence of paternal exposure to anaesthetics influencing the reproductive performance of the partners of nearly 8,000 male doctors.

A later study by Dr P. J. Tomlin of the University Department of Anaesthetics at Queen Elizabeth Hospital, Birmingham, showed that one in ten of the children born to anaesthetists in the West Midlands region had been referred to a consultant because of a congenital or non-acquired anomaly, most of which were concentrated in the central nervous system and musculoskeletal system, with girls apparently worst affected. Dr Tomlin's study, which covered 10 per cent of all anaesthetists in England and Wales, was publicized in the press and questions were asked in Parliament. It was also attacked as unduly alarmist by members of the team who carried out the study of 8,000 British male doctors and by Professor Sir Richard Doll, the Regius Professor of Medicine at Oxford University.

Professor Doll argued that Dr Tomlin's conclusion 'that employment as an anaesthetist involves an occupational hazard of cancer both for the anaesthetist and his or her children would be of grave concern if it were justified by the evidence. The evidence, however, is very frail. Dr Tomlin's data consist of 2 cases of cancer in 277 children of various ages up to twenty years and 2 cases of cancer of the breast at some time in the lives of seventy-six female anaesthetists. These numbers, he concludes, are respectively sixty and fifty times more than would be expected from national experience.' The comparison, Professor Doll argued, was inappropriate, since cumulative rates for the whole of the subjects' lives were being compared with national incidence rates for a single year.

Faced with a barrage of criticism and by what he called the 'cavalier treatment' of his results, Dr Tomlin retorted, 'Clearly, the question of health hazards arising out of pollution is an emotive subject; but resolution of this problem will not be helped by hyperbole, distortion, or mis-representation.' He also suggested that while the disputes about the statistics went on, 'at least one more child every month will be born with a congenital anomaly in an anaesthetist's family. This, of course, ignores the other workers in our operating theatres and their families.'

The relatively small number of problem cases involved in this controversy, as in some others, has meant that it has been hard to interpret the statistical data in a way which makes sense to all involved. Other studies, however, have proved beyond dispute that some other industrial chemicals are resulting in increased rates of abortion or miscarriage among women exposed to them. One Finnish research group analysed spontaneous abortions in relation to women's occupation using information on 11,731 such abortions, and found that there was a significant increase of spontaneous abortion in agricultural, industrial and construction workers, and a significant decrease in such office occupations as book-keeping. This study, however, did not control for such variables as drinking or smoking habits which, as we have seen, could significantly influence the results.

In a similar study of Finnish chemical workers, an increased spontaneous abortion rate was found, with some classes of workers at particular risk – including those involved in the plastics industry, in styrene production and use, and in the viscose rayon industry. As the Guy's Hospital Medical School team who reviewed this research pointed out, the type of analysis used 'cannot distinguish between chemical exposure and other occupationally related factors, such as nutrition, socio-economic status and so on. However, since the risk of spontaneous abortion was higher for chemical workers than for women employed in industry or construction trades, it suggests that chemical rather than socio-economic factors might be causally related to the risk.'

When a study of Finnish metal workers was undertaken it was found that the incidence of spontaneous abortions was not significantly higher than that for Finnish women as a whole, but it was significantly increased in the electronics sector and particularly among women involved in soldering operations. The radio and television production sectors stood out as problem areas.

Apart from the chemicals mentioned above, aniline, benzene, ethylene oxide, formaldehyde and lead have all been implicated to some degree in causing abortions or infertility. The evidence is indisputable against a chemical such as aniline, although there are uncertainties in some of the studies which have been published. We have already looked at the disruption of the menstrual cycle of some workers in the aniline dye industry in the western Urals and, perhaps not surprisingly, an increased abortion rate was also reported. Strangely, though, the highest incidence of spontaneous abortion was in a low-exposure area. When the investigators looked a little closer, they found that the work done in this area required a high degree of physical exertion, suggesting that there may have been a number of factors other than aniline exposure at work in producing the observed problems. But aniline is known to be implicated in the formation of methaemoglobin in the foetus, which lacks some of the enzymes needed to break down this material. Indeed, it has been recognized since 1886 that babies may become cyanosed (a condition in which the blood circulating through the skin lacks oxygen, giving the baby a bluish conplexion) if their nappies are stamped with aniline dyes.

Clearly, damage to the developing foetus in the womb is far from the only interest of reproductive toxicologists but, given the potential seriousness of the outcome of such damage, the period of pregnancy itself is considered in detail in the following chapter. Following the thalidomide disaster, and other incidents which showed that the mother's exposure to some chemicals could result in severe damage to the foetus, the field of teratology (the study of foetal malformation) was given an enormous boost. The range of potential teratogens is now such that they must be dealt with in a separate chapter.

For the moment, let's move on to the period after birth, to complete the spectrum of reproductive effects now being studied around the world. Worryingly, it is now thought that the exposure of the nursing infant to industrial chemicals in breast milk may, with some chemicals, be more hazardous than exposure of the foetus in the womb (or of adults) to the same chemicals.

The suggestion that mother's milk may now be polluted is clearly an emotive one, and perhaps easy to exaggerate for emotive effect, but research has shown that almost all foreign compounds that find their way into the blood of lactating women can also appear in breast milk. Most of the measurements of industrial chemicals in breast milk recorded in the literature have tended to be isolated measurements, which are certainly useful indicators of whether or not a particular chemical can be passed to the suckling infant in the milk, but reliable conclusions about the burden of such chemicals absorbed by the infant can only be reached where the measurements are related to a known exposure to a known chemical.

Some classes of industrial compound, the Guy's Hospital Medical School team reported, 'particularly those which are fat-soluble and water-soluble, are known to pass into the breast milk in significant quantities. Examples are the organohalides and for some of these, such as polychlorinated or polybrominated biphenyls, which are not broken down and persist in the body for very long periods of time, excretion via the breast milk may be the only major route of elimination from the body. Other industrial chemicals known to be selectively concentrated in the breast milk include pesticides such as chlordecone (Kepone), heptachlor epoxide, mirex, chlordane, aldrin, dieldrin, DDT and its metabolites, and the antifungal agent hexachlorobenzene.'

Polybrominated biphenyls (PBBs) have been involved in one of the worst cases of environmental contamination ever reported. If you live in the northern state of Michigan in the United States, it is highly likely that your blood and tissues are contaminated with PBBs – which are highly soluble in fat, are able to cross the placental barrier and indisputably appear in breast milk. In fact, newborn infants in a PBB-contaminated world are likely to absorb far more of this material while at their mother's breast than they ever did in the womb. Levels of PBB in human milk have been found to be about one hundred times higher than in the mother's plasma, suggesting that milk is a major excretion pathway for PBBs.

The Michigan PBB disaster has been described in great depth elsewhere, as in Joyce Egginton's excellent, if horrifying, book *Bitter Harvest*. The source of the poisoning was a mix-up at the Michigan Chemical Corporation which resulted in the mixing of very substantial quantities of Firemaster, a flame retardant, with a variety of cattle foods, including Nutrimaster. One version of the story has the Michigan Chemical Corporation running out of the red bag in which it shipped Firemaster and proceeding to pack it in the brown bags usually used for shipping Nutrimaster, with the inevitable mix-up duly happening.

Over 30,000 dairy cattle, 1.6 million chickens, 5 million eggs, and thousands of pigs and sheep had to be destroyed in an attempt to control the spread of the PBBs which were the principle ingredient in Firemaster, but the contaminated meat, dairy products, poultry and eggs already consumed over a period of nine months had spread the PBBs to such an extent that the majority (97 per cent) of the state's inhabitants (or eight to nine million people) showed measurable levels of PBBs in their blood and tissues.

Farmers and their families proved to be particularly at risk, with the 'PBB syndrome' proving to have some highly unfortunate implications for the state agricultural business. Apart from causing the destruction of staggering numbers of farm animals, the syndrome undermined the health of many whose health was utterly indispensable to their livelihood. To take just one effect, many workers who had previously only needed six to seven hours of sleep a night found that they needed sixteen to eighteen after the accident.

When the Mount Sinai School of Medicine, New York, launched a study of chronic PBB contamination in Michigan some five years after the event, tissue samples taken from 844 subjects showed PBB levels up to 36 parts per million, with a mean value of 0.4 parts per million. And blood from another 1,681 adults and children showed that 70 per cent of them were contaminated, although at much lower levels – of about 1 to 2 parts per billion. This contamination proved to be worse in the children and men, perhaps because the children had been drinking more contaminated milk while men have less body fat than women, so that a given dose will be concentrated in fewer fat cells.

The first full report on the affected herds in Michigan appeared in 1974 and showed that a large number of cows which had been artificially inseminated had come back into oestrus within four to six weeks. Indeed, it was suspected that the embryos were being re-absorbed by the cows, although this could not at that time be confirmed. A wide range of reproductive effects in cattle were reported over the ensuing years, including late births, stillbirths and early deaths among the resulting calves.

One of the most worrying aspects of what Joyce Egginton later decribed as 'probably the most widespread and least reported chemical disaster ever to happen in the western world', was that 'all the relevant institutions of democracy failed. Rather than working together for the public good they operated, individually and collectively, against it – not out of malice, but simply because this was an event outside their experience and beyond their budgetary means to resolve. The state agencies underestimated the seriousness of the situation and, when they finally acknowledged it, tried to cover their earlier inadequacies. The governor of Michigan took his advice from the state agencies, and more than two years passed before he realized he had been misled. Various departments of the federal government decided that, since the contamination was confined to Michigan, it was not their responsibility. Although an entire state was affected, it could not be designated a federal disaster area, entitled to relief funds, because the disaster was not one of nature's excesses but the result of an industrial accident for which industry should compensate. The aggrieved were left to seek redress through the legal system, where they were out-matched by the superior resources of those corporate giants whose employees – through carelessness and human error – were responsible for poisoning their bodies and their land.'

Worryingly, similar effects have been reported in dairy herds in Ireland and Scotland. In both cases, government surveys cleared the industrial plants which had been accused of causing these effects, but in the case of Re-Chem International's waste incineration plant at Bonnybridge, Scotland, the controversy proved to be the last straw. The plant, Re-Chem said when announcing its closure, had been running at a loss for years.

In fact the Bonnybridge controversy was a prime example of some of the paradoxes which often surface in such cases. Some environmentalists, for example, argued vigorously in Re-Chem's favour, pointing out that if the plant closed the industrial wastes, including PCBs, which were previously incinerated there, could well end up elsewhere, causing 'wholesale, unregulated pollution of the environment'. And the farmer who had laid the charges against Re-Chem had been refusing to allow independent vets or pollution experts onto his land. Such cases are almost tailor-made to generate heat rather than to cast light on major pollution issues. Indeed, the controversy really took off when a Canadian scientist, Dr Brock Chittam, found about one part per billion of dioxin in a soil sample given to him by the farmer. Even so, it was far from clear whether the dioxin had come from the Re-Chem plant, which the various pollution control authorities had never detected putting out dioxin. And, even if the dioxin *had* come from the plant, it was by no means the only possible cause of the cattle diseases reported.

Interestingly, as Joyce Egginton pointed out, 'PBB came under intense investigation because of the cattle feed contamination. Otherwise, like hundreds of other synthetic organic compounds which are created every year, it would have escaped public attention. It was never a widely used chemical. Although it had been around for three years before the misshipment from Michigan Chemical Corporation, most chemists had never heard of it.'

Having spent three years studying what she dubbed the 'ultimate experiment', she concluded that 'the research which has been done on PBB would fill a fat textbook, and the careful reader would find a moral in it: the more that chemists try to analyze this – or any other similar compound – the more they realize how little they understand. Because of the Michigan accident, at least nine million people have PBB in their systems. But because of the way in which our world has developed, everyone living in an indus-trialized society has accumulated a peculiarly personal combina-tion of chemical residues which may, or may not, eventually cause harm. Nobody knows whether some of these cancel others out, or whether, reacting to different metabolisms and genetic make-ups, their combined effect is additive, antagonistic, or synergistic. Given all these unknowns,' she stressed, 'the accepted concept of a standard "tolerance level" for any contaminant becomes mean-ingless.'

Work is under way in many research institutions to develop new genetic screening techniques, to identify those who may be particularly susceptible to exposure to particular chemicals, but the evaluation of the long-term health and reproductive effects of the multiple exposures to chemicals which are part and parcel of present-day life in an industrial society are another matter altogether.

Before leaving the PBB disaster, it is worth noting that despite this vast, unplanned 'ultimate experiment', the amount of reliable data available about the reproductive effects of PBBs in people is still surprisingly small. When the Guy's Hospital Medical School team looked at the evidence on PBBs, it concluded that there was clear evidence, in animal studies at least, that PBBs could be toxic at low levels both in the early stages of the reproductive cycle and during pregnancy itself. A number of studies had been carried out on animals to check the material's carcinogenicity and muta-genicity, but the conclusion drawn was that the resulting data were 'inadequate for evaluation'. But the possibility that PBBs can act as carcinogens in humans is still wide open – with another twenty-five to thirty years needed before anyone will be able to write the final chapter on this particular incident.

A carcinogen's effects can emerge considerably earlier, if it can act as a 'transplacental carcinogen' – passing through the placenta during pregnancy and causing cancers either in the foetus or, more probably, in the developing children after birth. Only one such agent, the drug diethylstilboestrol (DES), has been conclusively identified in humans, and its history is discussed further in

Chapter 4. But animal studies have shown that most chemical carcinogens can also act transplacentally and that the developing foetus is typically more sensitive to such agents than are adults.

Again, some industries emerge as more of a problem than others. When the University of Southern California Medical School took ninety-two children with brain tumours and checked the occupational exposure of their parents, ten of the children proved to have fathers working in the aircraft industry around Los Angeles. Among the control group of ninety-two families picked from the same neighbourhoods, none reported a parent working in the aircraft industry.

If the results of this study were extrapolated to the United States as a whole, according to Dr John M. Peters, who led the study team, it could mean that chemical exposure of parents accounts for 25 per cent of all childhood brain tumours – which are the second most serious cause of cancer death among children, after leukaemia.

The study, which was the first to show a relationship between such tumours and the occupation of parents, found a seven times greater workplace exposure to paint fumes and a three times greater exposure to chemical solvents among fathers of diseased children than among fathers in the control group. It also found that the mothers of such children reported a three times greater exposure to chemicals than did mothers in the control group. Dr Peters commented that the tumours could have resulted either from genetic damage caused in the father's reproductive system or, more directly, from chemicals clinging to the father's clothing when he returned from work.

It would be interesting to know whether similar effects have emerged among the children of workers in the new semiconductor industry, the general safety record of which has been above average. Meanwhile, whatever effects may emerge from such unintentional environmental exposures, clear evidence has emerged to show that intentional exposures, or at least exposures where the mother intentionally exposed herself to the suspected chemical, can cause childhood cancers.

It has been estimated, for example, that about 250 of the 1,200 or so childhood cancers which develop each year in British children aged up to fifteen could be caused by drugs which their mothers took during pregnancy. The comments which follow, however, need to be prefaced by an indication of the relatively small risks of childhood cancer found in the population as a whole. In Britain, the risk of a baby being born with cancer or developing cancer in later childhood is about 1 in 1,000, compared to a 1-in-500 risk of mongolism (or Down's syndrome) and a 1-in-200 risk of spina bifida or of anencephaly (where the baby is born without all or part of the brain). Clearly, we are not talking about a plague, and many of the drugs which may prove to cause occasional cancers are taken by large numbers of women with no observable adverse effect.

That said, a Birmingham-based research group has laboriously collected information on every child who has died of cancer in England, Scotland and Wales since the early 1950s. The research group, which is located in Birmingham University's Department of Community Medicine, is officially known as the Oxford Survey of Childhood Cancer because its work, later taken over by Professor George Knox of Birmingham, was originally begun by Dr Alice Stewart at Oxford University. The data the group has collected are now so voluminous that it may well be able to pinpoint unsuspected links between certain drugs, and even certain brands of drug, and the incidence of childhood cancers.

For a long time it was thought that chemicals were not a threat during pregnancy because the placenta was seen as an infallible screen. Now, with problems such as those caused by diethylstilbestrol (DES) and thalidomide in mind, it is obvious that this view was mistaken. Following the DES saga, the Birmingham group began to sift through the list of hormones and other drugs given in pregnancy to see if any might cause childhood cancers. Strangely, they failed to find evidence that hormones could cause transplacental cancers, although this may simply be because DES was less widely used in Britain than it was in the United States and because the girls in the group's sample were still too young to develop the vaginal cancer which is the hallmark of DES.

But the group's evidence had begun to incriminate a number of other drugs. The data for 1972–7, for example, show that the mothers of the 2,707 children who died of cancer during that period were significantly more likely to have taken sleeping tablets, tranquillizers or antibiotics during pregnancy. While the suggestion is that some of these may be implicated in childhood cancers, it is also possible that some of the cancers may have been caused by viral infections or other problems for which the suspect drugs were prescribed.

Sedatives, however, have come under suspicion because it is thought that some such drugs may depress a child's ability to break down chemicals which may cause cancer. As Professor Knox has put it, 'Pregnant rats given very small doses of certain chemicals called nitrosamines have offspring which develop cancer in a highly predictable way.' Such carcinogens are typically broken down in the liver into harmless (or less harmful) substances. Then researchers at Cornell University, New York, found that if the sedative drug phenobarbital was given to female rats while they were suckling their young, these young were highly likely to show massive liver damage. The drug, it was discovered, was reaching the young rats through their mothers' milk and blocking or suppressing the enzymatic processes by which they would normally inactivate cancer-causing agents. The implication, clearly, is that some drugs to which young animals are exposed, either in the womb or during breast-feeding, may increase the risk of cancer.

Another type of pollution effect, and it is one which has been much investigated in relation to lead pollution, involves changes in the process of brain development, which continues for about two years after the birth of a child. But the problem with so many of these possible effects is that once a group of people, including foetuses and children, has been exposed to a chemical, those responsible for tracking any health effects may find that there are all sorts of confounding considerations to be taken into account. If, on the other hand, they decide to set up a controlled trial in humans, the chances are that they will never get their study off the ground. The fierce controversy which surrounded proposed trials in Britain, designed to discover whether vitamin supplements given to mothers might reduce the incidence of spina bifida, is a case in point.

The original intention was to launch a five-year, £300,000, experimental programme involving at least 2,000 women who had already given birth to a child suffering from spina bifida or a related defect and who wished to have another child. In 1981, 663 spina bifida babies were born in England and Wales, and the question in the minds of the research team was whether the use of such vitamin supplements as folic acid could help prevent the disease even in susceptible mothers.

Consider the Medical Research Council's view of the matter. It is known, for example, that the brain and spinal cord of the developing embryo first form as a long flat strip, which folds to form a cylinder some three to four weeks after conception. In a few cases in a thousand, this process goes wrong and the result may be a spina bifida baby. The cause of the disorder is not known, although it is known that the incidence of the disease varies from country to country and from area to area, as well as varying by the season of the year and the social class of the mother. Mothers who have already had one affected child are ten times more likely to have another. Two studies had suggested that folic acid given before and around conception can reduce the risk, but the Medical Research Council concluded that 'the evidence so far obtained, though suggestive, remains so inconclusive that it does not justify offering extra vitamins to all women at risk. The extra vitamins themselves,' it noted, 'may not be without risks and some of their functions are still incompletely understood.'

The Council's view was that the only way to settle the issue was to set up a large-scale clinical trial in which, to avoid bias, women at risk would be randomly allocated to various forms of treatment, including a control treatment – that is, one lacking the vitamin supplements. Although the Council said a woman taking part in the trials would be entered only by consent and after all the relevant considerations had been explained to her by her doctor, the implication that some women would be denied potentially effective treatment was not well received.

Yet the use of control groups is essential if such research is to produce meaningful results. It is also vitally important that these control groups be carefully matched, to exclude possible confounding factors such as age, dietary intake, and any smoking or drinking habits.

A number of the problems and disorders discussed above occur naturally, including infertility, menstrual disorders and disruptions of spontaneous abortions – indeed one can say they are fairly common. If isolated cases of such reproductive effects emerge, it is difficult to make very much of them, since they are almost certainly related to natural causes; but if small clusters of reported problems begin to appear in one place, the warning bells should sound. One problem chemical, dibromochloropropane, was tracked down after a group of workers discovered during an everyday conversation that a number of them had become infertile.

Often, it appears, such effects are discovered almost by chance.

It was discovered that one group of farm workers which included four cases of impotence was adversely affected by exposure to a range of pesticides and herbicides while working on one estate only when three of the men attended the same local doctor – who was the first person to recognize that a link might exist.

Another problematic area is where the chemical under suspicion has only a small effect. As the Guy's Hospital Medical School team put it, 'to detect a doubling in frequency of a congenital malformation such as anencephaly, with a background spontaneous incidence of one in 1,000 live births, a total of 23,000 live births in exposed persons would need to be studied. Even then, there would still be a 5 per cent chance of missing a genuine effect. Clearly, few studies will be of sufficient size to exclude the possibility of such small effects.'

Reproductive toxicity, however rare or difficult to pinpoint the effects may be, is often a particularly sensitive indicator of a chemical's toxicity – and the results of such research are obviously of considerable interest to anyone exposed to or likely to be exposed to such chemicals. Given the psychological aspects of some reproductive effects, such as menstrual disorders and sexual libido or potency, it may be difficult to interpret some of the effects discussed above. But other aspects of the human reproductive cycle, such as sperm counts, numbers of live and still births, birth weights, and infant survival and malformation rates, can be reliable indicators of a chemical's toxicity or teratogenicity (ability to cause birth defects).

Life before birth is the subject of the next chapter, together with the environmental challenges which the foetus must overcome if it is to be born at all. The picture of life in the womb as the ultimate idyll is itself under challenge. The unborn, it emerges, join our industrial societies far sooner than most of us had imagined. Like the fish which swim through unseen worlds on the other side of our effluent outfalls, the foetus no longer lives in an unpolluted sea.

THE
PLACENTA
BETRAYED

If we think about it at all, most of us tend to think of the womb as the Eden from which we were so rudely expelled at birth. We picture the foetus enjoying the 'ultimate idyll', as Geraldine Youcha put it recently. 'Clean, serene, protected from noxious substances by the complex filtering system of the placenta, shielded from the jolts, noise and stress of the world a few inches away, the fetus sleeps. Cradled in warm fluid, blissfully insensate, it floats cozily until it is thrust into the atmosphere and its brain, eyes and ears switch on for the first time.'

But science, which has robbed us of other reassuring illusions, such as the idea that the sun revolves around our home planet or the belief that our species has remained unchanged since it was created just over 4,000 years ago by divine intervention, has increasingly challenged this comfortable view of life before birth. We have already seen that the sperm, the egg and the fertilized egg must overcome certain chemical hurdles before successful implantation in the uterine wall is achieved – and there is now a growing body of evidence proving beyond doubt that the twentieth-century womb itself can be a very much more inhospitable place than one might expect.

Some of the threats to the unborn are perfectly natural, seeming to be a twentieth-century problem simply because twentieth-century technology has enabled us to identify and study them for the first time. An example of this is the phenomenon of the

'vanishing twin' which first really came to light with the development of ultrasound scanning techniques. With ultrasound, doctors
can 'see' into the womb and identify multiple pregnancies very
much earlier than hitherto. Having done so, they found that a
surprising number of pregnancies which they had initially diagnosed as multiple pregnancies were turning out to be conventional
single pregnancies. What, they wondered, was going on?

The answer was totally unexpected. There was no fault in the
scanning technology: multiple pregnancies were being correctly
identified as such. It transpired that the human embryo, like the
embryos of many other mammals, can be reabsorbed into the
mother's tissue. Obstetricians Louis Keith and Helain Landy of
Northwestern University Medical School in the USA combed the
medical literature to check the frequency of vanishing twin cases.
They concluded that even with ultrasound many early foetal re-
absorptions are missed – and that between 10 and 20 per cent of
all twins conceived can vanish during gestation. There are those
who believe that this estimate is very much on the low side. In one
study of pregnant women, Salvatore Levi of Brugman University
Hospital in Brussels found that of those mothers initially found to
be carrying twins, an astonishing 71 per cent ultimately gave birth
to a single infant.

It is still far from clear how the process actually happens, but it
seems that something in the foetal environment selects the hardier
of two or more womb-mates for survival. As Dr Keith put it, 'In
many of our reproductive functions, we are no different from other
animals except for the fact that we don't have litters. But maybe
we *do* have litters. Maybe human beings have multiple fertiliza-
tions much more commonly than we ever believed.'

A great deal goes on in the womb which most of us never even
suspected, largely because we never gave it a thought. But even
in those areas where we actually thought we did know something
concrete about the foetal environment, we now find that our basic
assumptions are being undermined. One very recent field of
investigation, for instance, is prenatal psychology, with many
research studies beginning to suggest that the foetus is not a
mindless, insensate assembly of organs waiting for birth to turn
them on. Instead, it appears, the foetus can see, hear, taste and
even learn, in a very primitive way, *in utero* – that is, in the womb
– before birth.

Thomas Verny, who has concluded that the emotional make-up of the unborn child can be affected and shaped during gestation by the behaviour and emotions of its mother, points out that many ancient cultures believed that the mother's experiences during pregnancy could influence the unborn child, for good or ill. And as for the notion that the foetus is totally insulated from external events while in the womb, Dr Verny has found many references in such texts as Hippocrates' journals and the Bible which suggest exactly the opposite. He quotes St Luke 1:44, where Elizabeth exclaims, 'For lo, as soon as the voice of thy salutation sounded in mine ears, the babe leaped in my womb for joy.' Dr Henry Truby, as Professor of Paediatrics, Linguistics and Anthropology at the University of Miami, found that the foetus can hear clearly from the sixth month – and that it moves its body in rhythm with its mother's speech.

Another assumption that has been challenged, and horribly so, in recent years is that the placenta is impregnable to external assault. Far from it. Chemicals absorbed or ingested by the mother all cross the placental barrier to some extent whether they be taken for therapeutic reasons (as in the case of medicinal drugs), for recreational reasons (as with the drinking of alcohol, smoking or the use of hallucinogenic drugs) or inadvertently, as in the case of some food additives and all forms of environmental pollution. Some, such as methyl mercury, are preferentially concentrated in the foetus, while others may largely (but not entirely) be kept at bay by the placenta.

We still have a fair amount to learn about the placenta, which is emerging as a far more extraordinary organ than anyone had suspected. 'The placenta is often thought to be little more than an attachment for an umbilical cord that like a diver's air hose conveys oxygen to the fetus growing in the amniotic fluid that fills the pregnant uterus,' concluded one team of British physicians which focused its attention on the placenta for many years. Based at University College London, Professor Peter Beaconsfield's team pointed out that the placenta, 'rather than serving as a passive filter, is both active and selective in its transfer of substances essential to the development of the fetus'. It can also be an active and selective filter where the transfer of substances which are likely to be injurious to foetal health is concerned.

The placenta is certainly an extraordinary organ. Few of us realize that both the placenta and the foetus derive from the same single cell: the fertilized ovum. The significance of the umbilical cord, which connects placenta and foetus, has long been recognized. Indeed, the barber's pole and the Aesculapian staff of life are both thought to have been inspired by the red veins which spiral round the white cord. 'Yet little attention, symbolic or otherwise, has been paid to the placenta,' the UCL team stressed, 'without which the cord would have nothing to supply and without which the fetus could not grow. The umbilical cord delivers far more than oxygen to the fetus, and the placenta does far more than simply anchor the cord. Thickly supplied with fetal blood vessels on one side and washed with maternal blood on the other, the placenta anatomically separates the circulatory systems of the fetus and the mother, so that all exchanges of material in any form must take place across this interface. During its brief life span the placenta is therefore the sole purveyor of all fetal needs and the sole route of disposal for all fetal wastes.'

The successive stages of the placenta's development are illustrated in Figures 4.1–4.7. Researchers, including those in the UCL team, have been fascinated by the way in which the placenta grows, acting in many respects like a tumour, and invades the maternal uterine tissue. Once the placenta has implanted itself, the blastocyst cells from which the embryo develops – and then the foetus and placenta – are parasitic on the mother, becoming totally dependent on her for oxygen, fluids, nutrients, salts and hormones. But the relationship between the mother and her developing child, a two-way relationship which is 'switched' through the placenta in much the same way that telephone calls need to be routed through an exchange, is infinitely more complex than this analogy might suggest.

The placenta is at once a protein factory and a power plant, synthesizing many of the proteins needed to build the foetus and generating the energy needed to integrate them within the rapidly developing foetal structure. This activity proceeds at a very much greater volume and pace than in any other organ, as the UCL team pointed out, because 'the placenta must not only itself grow but also serve as a builder's yard and power plant for a fetus that will rapidly outgrow it several times over'.

There is still a great deal we do not know about the ways in which the invading placenta, along with its villous projections, manages to avoid triggering the mother's immune response. But some facts are incontrovertible: human placentas may vary in size,

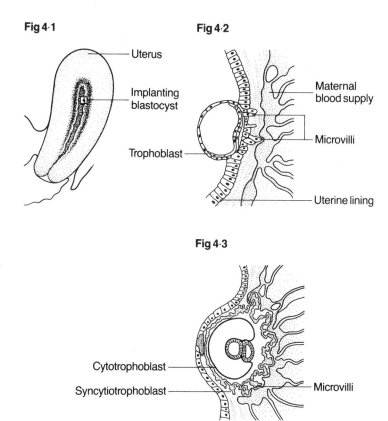

Fig 4·1

- Uterus
- Implanting blastocyst
- Trophoblast

Fig 4·2

- Maternal blood supply
- Microvilli
- Uterine lining

Fig 4·3

- Cytotrophoblast
- Syncytiotrophoblast
- Microvilli

Figure 4.1–4.7 In a normal pregnancy, the foetus and the placenta which sustains it develop in tandem, as illustrated in Figures 4.1–4.7. The process begins with the implantation of the fertilized egg (blastocyst) in the wall of the uterus. As the blastocyst makes contact with the uterine lining (endometrium) the layer of cells (trophoblast) which will develop into the placenta begins to send finger-like projections (microvilli) into the endometrial lining – as illustrated in Figures 4.2 and 4.3. During this invasive stage, the trophoblast and the developing foetus are linked by the body stalk, which later evolves into the umbilical cord, as is shown in Figures 4.4–4.7.

By the time birth is imminent, the placenta is a large, disc-shaped structure. It is typically about 20 centimetres in diameter and some 3 centimetres deep in the middle. The average placenta at birth weighs some 500 grams, or approximately one sixth of the weight of the infant it has nurtured. (*Source*: Beaconsfield, Birdwood and Beaconsfield, *Scientific American*, August 1980, pp. 94–102)

Fig 4·4

Fig 4·5

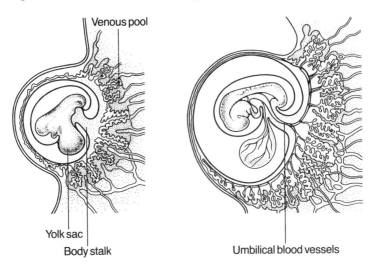

Venous pool

Yolk sac

Body stalk

Umbilical blood vessels

Fig 4·6

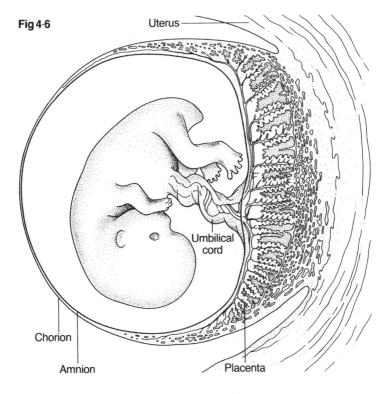

Uterus

Umbilical cord

Chorion

Amnion

Placenta

Fig 4·7

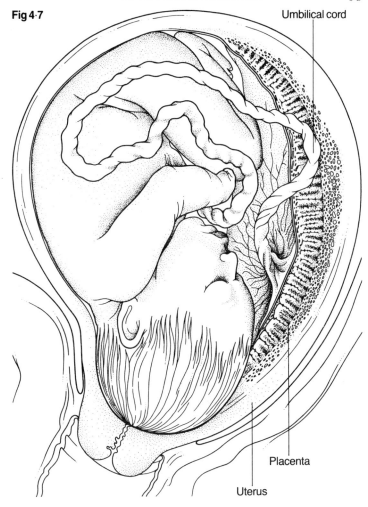

Umbilical cord

Placenta

Uterus

shape and weight, but when the average child is born it is about six times heavier than the placenta which nurtured it for the previous nine months. Anyone who has seen this protein factory after a birth will recall a disc-shaped object weighing perhaps 500 grams and having a diameter of perhaps 20 centimetres. Typically it is up to 3 centimetres thick in its central area, tapering off towards the edges. Yet no other organ in the human body carries out the synthesis of such a tremendous array of proteins for such a wide spectrum of purposes.

Contrary to most people's expectations, relatively little of the raw material which the placenta extracts from the massive flow of blood from the mother's system is received in the form in which it is needed for foetal and placental development. So, while the placenta must simultaneously serve as a sorting, processing and production facility for the protein building-blocks it needs for its own construction and operation, it must also keep up with the pace and range of foetal demands. The placenta's metabolic rate is prodigious: by the tenth week after fertilization, when the placenta weighs about 50 grams (or 10 per cent of its ultimate weight), it should be producing about 1.5 grams of protein every day, rising to about 7.5 grams a day by the time birth is imminent.

The placenta uses about a third of all the oxygen and glucose supplied to it to fuel its own metabolism, a metabolism which involves the production of many of the hormones which most of us who have never given the process much thought would have assumed were produced by the mother. Indeed, from the earliest days of pregnancy, the cells of the trophoblast and its placental successors manufacture an astonishing variety of hormones. One of the first to be produced in significant quantities is the protein hormone chorionic gonadotrophin, which appears to be used as a protective immunological coating around the outer cell surfaces of the trophoblast, preventing the maternal rejection of the blastocyst.

In laboratory experiments, many of the substances produced by the placenta have proved able to suppress the activity of lymphocytes, the cells which would normally promote the rejection of a tissue graft (which is what the placenta effectively is), including human chorionic gonadotrophin, placental lactogen and prolactin, the steroid hormones cortisone, progesterone and the oestrogens, and a range of other proteins and glycoproteins. In fact, some scientists believe that tumours are pathological tissues which have 'understood' and exploited some of the placenta's ruses to prevent their own rejection by the host tissue.

However that may be, there is no doubting the exquisite versatility of the placenta in coping with the changing needs of the developing foetus. A single example of this versatility and close-tuning comes from work carried out by Dr Dorothy Villee of the Harvard Medical School on the synthesis of steroid hormones in the placenta. As the UCL team explained it, 'The human placenta lacks the enzymes needed for converting the large amounts of progesterone it makes into certain essential estrogens and other steroids. Dr Villee has found that the synthesis of these hormones from progesterone is carried out in "fetal zone" cells: clusters of transient cells found in the developing adrenal glands of the fetus that lack the enzymes necessary to manufacture progesterone but possess the requisite ones for its conversion. In this way the fetal and placental tissues complement each other. In fact, some of the "fetal" estrogen even returns to the placenta for further manipulation.'

By producing this array of hormones, the placenta not only stands in for the foetal pituitary gland until that organ is ready to perform on its own but also 'conducts the entire endocrine orchestra of pregnancy, which performs largely in the placenta itself'.

Before turning to look at some of the problems which can arise when the human placenta plugs into the twentieth century, it is worth looking briefly at the world from the foetus's point of view. When the human egg is fertilized, it is about the size of a full stop on this page – and the sperm is 20,000 times smaller. Five weeks after fertilization, the embryo is about 10 millimetres long, its brain has begun to develop, and its heart is already pumping blood through the placenta and around its own body. At this stage, it is worth noting, the embryo is under 1.5 cm long – less than half the length of a standard paper-clip.

After two months, the embryo is recognizably human, is nearly 6 centimetres long (or as long as $2\frac{1}{2}$ paper-clips laid end to end), has forelimbs with fingers and toes, and already has a well formed face. From this stage on, the embryo is called a foetus. By the sixth month of pregnancy, the embryo is almost 30 centimetres long, has hair, finger-nails and toe-nails, and its milk teeth are developing in its jaws. At birth, a baby typically weighs between 3 and 3.5 kilograms and has reached a length of about 50 centimetres.

The umbilical lifeline carries an artery and a vein from the embryo's circulatory system, blood vessels which plug into an immense network of capillaries extending throughout the placental disc and into the millions of finger-like villi which have grown into the uterine wall. These capillaries carry blood from the embryo to within a fraction of a millimetre of the maternal blood supply, so that oxygen and nutrients can diffuse across from the mother's

blood into that of the embryo, while carbon dioxide and
nitrogenous wastes diffuse out of the embryo's blood and into the
maternal bloodstream.

The placenta thus *does* serve as a filter, given that the mother's
blood never, under normal circumstances, flows into the embryo.
But, as we shall see, it is far from infallible in this particular task.
Indeed, a pollutant like methyl mercury may be preferentially
concentrated in the embryo or foetus by means of a process described on p. 113, with the pollutant encouraged to cross the
placental barrier and the embryo or foetus trapping the pollutant
almost like a magnet attracting iron filings.

There are three broad stages in the development of a foetus at
which it may be exposed to external threats: during fertilization
and implantation, during the embryonic stage (up to about two
months after fertilization) and during the foetal stage itself. The
significance of any injury depends very much on when it takes
place. If it occurs during the period of fertilization and implantation, which spans from conception to seventeen days into pregnancy, cells in the blastocyst may be damaged or even killed.
However, since all cells are still 'totipotent', able to adopt any role
in the following stages of development, the clump of cells can
recover and continue to multiply. If this happens, then the embryo
should show no structural deformities later in its development.
Alternatively, the injury may be lethal to the blastocyst, resulting
either in early abortion or in reabsorption into the mother's tissue.

The next stage, the embryonic period, lasts from day 18 to day
55 – and turns out to be by far the most critical period in the
transition from a fertilized egg to a newborn child. This is the period
during which the mass of undifferentiated cells in the blastocyst
start to begin to develop into distinct organs, a process called
organogenesis. Each organ system differentiates at a different rate
and has its own critical period of development. If the embryo is
exposed to a teratogen, an agent able to induce birth defects, the
nature of the resulting defects will very much depend on the critical
periods with which the teratogenic exposure coincides.

The third, foetal, stage is very much less sensitive to such challenges, although it is far from immune to environmental threats.
From day 56 to birth, however, any agent which does not directly
kill the foetus tends to influence cell size and number. Consequently, growth retardation or injury to the central nervous

system are most likely to result from any toxic exposures during this phase of development. The brain remains vulnerable, since its development (including myelination, the process by which the larger nerve fibres are sheathed with such substances as phospholipid and cholesterol) is still incomplete at birth.

Birth defects go back beyond the dawn of time, a varying combination of genetic and environmental factors contributing to their occurrence in animal populations and in the populations of preindustrial societies. Usually the birth of a deformed child was regarded as a tragedy, although very occasionally it was seen as a sign from the gods and the deformed child treated as a god in its own right. In Egypt, for example, a number of mummified deformed children have been found, adorned as gods.

If the hand of the local god or gods was not suspected, then the deformity was sometimes seen as an indication that astrological influences were at work, and that perhaps the position of the appropriate star or planet had been awry at the time of conception. Another possible explanation, as Dr John Tesh of Life Science Research has pointed out, involved hybridization with animals. 'Any abnormal child that was born with any feature resembling an animal was thought to be due to bestiality, with the mother having had sexual relations with an animal,' Dr Tesh explained, 'even in the most unlikely combinations: for example, the development of a proboscis was attributed to relations with an elephant; the fusion of the lower limbs, as in sirenomelia or "mermaid"-type deformities, was attributed to relations with a large fish.' And another class of 'explanations' for birth defects attributed them to something the mother saw during pregnancy. 'Many types of visual impression were thought to cause deformities in unborn children,' Dr Tesh told a group of Japanese toxicologists. 'Even up to a few years ago in country districts in Britain there was a strong belief that cleft lip, or hare-lip as it was known, was caused by the mother having seen a hare during her pregnancy.'

Various cultures developed various ways of dealing with the problem: in many, pregnant women were cloistered to prevent their seeing anything untoward; in some, the birth of a deformed child was tackled by the horrible expedient of publicly executing both mother and child.

Today it is generally thought that there are four main classes of environmental teratogen: radiation, viruses, drugs and chemicals. Teratology, which has been probably the fastest growing area of concern within reproductive toxicology, itself probably the fastest growing area in toxicology, involves the study of the causes and development of disabling or lethal birth defects and congenital malformations that are present at birth – or appear soon after. The defect may be functional, involving the lack of an arm or leg; histological, involving the absence of (or defects in) a particular tissue; or biochemical, involving, for example, an inability to synthesize a particular enzyme.

The rapid advance of technology across an increasingly broad front has introduced very large numbers of new drugs, chemicals and other environmental agents, some of which have proved to be teratogenic. Strangely, while the old superstitions about the causes of birth defects were eroded, the idea that some of these new agents could have an impact on the unborn child was slow to take root. This situation continued through the 1940s and 1950s, despite the fact that embryologists, experimental anatomists and morphologists were publishing the results of work on experimental animals which suggested that foetal abnormalities could result from exposure to such agents as vitamin A, X-irradiation and trypan blue. Despite these findings, as Dr Tesh has put it, 'There seemed to be an almost naïve belief that the human foetus was completely immune from interference by drugs and chemicals.'

The consensus was that the placenta served as a very good barrier against such agents. 'It came as a tremendous shock,' Dr Tesh recalls, 'world wide, when it was realized that thalidomide had had such disastrous effects on the developing foetus.' First synthesized in 1954 by a Swiss pharmaceutical company which wanted to find new sedatives, thalidomide proved to have no significant sedative effect on experimental animals and was discarded. Next it was taken up by a West German company, Chemie Grünenthal, which ran up against the same problem. However, since the structure of the molecule strongly suggested that it should work as a sedative, Chemie Grünenthal tried it as an anticonvulsant for epileptics. It failed to prevent epileptic convulsions, but worked as a hypnotic drug, promoting deep sleep. The company thought that it had struck gold.

During 1960, under the trade name Contergan, it became the favourite sleeping tablet in West Germany, available cheaply and without a prescription. It turned out to be as safe for humans as for animals, with would-be suicides surviving large doses without apparent harm. As Helen Taussig, Professor of Paediatrics at the

Johns Hopkins School of Medicine, reported a couple of years later, the company 'combined thalidomide with aspirin and other medicines. Germans consumed these compounds for such conditions as colds, coughs, nervousness, neuralgia, migraine, and other headaches and asthma. A liquid form made especially for children became West Germany's baby-sitter. Hospitals employed it to quiet children for electro-encephalographic studies. As an anti-emetic, it helped to combat the nausea of pregnancy, and of course Contergan gave many a pregnant woman a good night's sleep. Grünenthal was manufacturing it almost by the ton.'

Soon the drug was being licensed to manufacturers in other countries, including Distillers (Biochemical Company) Ltd, which sold it as Distival in Britain, Australia and New Zealand. In Canada, it was marketed as Talimol and as Kevadon. In September 1960, the Wm S. Merrell Company of Cincinnati applied to the US Food and Drug Administration for clearance to sell Kevadon in the US market. Dr Frances Oldham Kelsey of the Food and Drug Administration is generally credited with stopping that application in its tracks.

The company, in fact, intended to recommend thalidomide for pregnant women, to combat nausea. Dr Kelsey insisted on data showing that the drug was safe if used during pregnancy, because she was convinced that the foetus, in pharmacological terms, is quite different from an adult. It was, and still is, extremely difficult to obtain reliable advance data on possible human teratogens by using experimental animals. Indeed, early tests on thalidomide proved contradictory, even after there was real suspicion about the drug's side-effects. The Grünenthal laboratories, for example, tried unsuccessfully to reproduce the thalidomide syndrome in rats, mice and rabbits, although it was shown that thalidomide could cross the placenta. Yet when Dr George Somers, as Distillers' pharmacologist, fed massive doses of the drug to pregnant rabbits, he found he had reproduced the worse effects of the thalidomide syndrome almost exactly.

Dr Somers, in fact, emerged from the resulting scandal with more than a clean slate. Early in 1959, he had found that a liquid preparation of the drug was definitely toxic, a finding which undermined his own company's claim that thalidomide was totally non-toxic. Dr Somers tried hard to get Distillers to publish his latest findings, which ran counter to his earlier conclusion that there appeared to be no lethal dose for thalidomide. 'Some day,' he told the company's senior management, 'someone is going to make the observations we have made with different formulations of thalidomide. They may publish them and cause us some damage. If we have already drawn attention to these matters,' he advised, 'we will be in a much stronger position.'

The company was not persuaded, choosing instead to keep this potentially damaging information under wraps. But by this time the medical journals were beginning to carry reports of a new polyneuritis associated with long-term use of thalidomide, with patients complaining of tingling hands, sensory disturbances and, later, motor disturbances and even atrophy of the thumb. By April 1961, there were a sufficient number of such reports for West Germany to place thalidomide compounds on the list of compounds for which a prescription was required; but they remained in widespread use.

The roadblock which the drug had hit in the United States proved particularly problematic, since Grünenthal had not carried out teratogenic tests on thalidomide before placing it on the market. Despite sales literature suggesting that the drug had been tested on pregnant women, this was not the case. When the *Sunday Times* Insight team wrote the book of their campaign against the thalidomide companies, they confirmed that 'Grünenthal, in order to sell its drug, thought it useful to give the impression that a clinical trial with pregnant women had been made. That certainly strengthened the "hypothesis of safety" as publicly perceived. Had Grünenthal actually thought to have such a trial conducted, and had it been competently organized, it would have been very likely that teratogenic effects could have been picked up with suffering confined to a dozen cases or so. But Grünenthal not only failed to conduct a clinical trial to examine thalidomide's safety in pregnancy, it failed as well to carry out any reproductive studies on animals.'

The company's response to this accusation had been that such tests were most unusual at the time. Not so, the Insight team retorted. 'It was in no way unusual for reproductive studies to be made with drugs in the days before thalidomide was invented, though practice varied among companies and, of course, among different drugs. There would be no point in doing reproductive studies with a drug designed to combat the effects of senility,' they accepted. 'But the scientific record makes it clear that many scientists considered that drugs in the sedative/hypnotic/tranquillizer bracket should be checked for reproductive dangers.'

When the first deformities began to appear, it was far from clear that thalidomide was to blame. The malformations were found to be fairly consistent, although they varied considerably in severity. The main class of deformity involved abnormalities in the long bones of the arms, with the legs also involved in about half the cases. The development of the human embryo from the third week to the eighth week is illustrated in Figures 4.8–4.13, while some thalidomide symptoms are shown in Figure 4.14. The first signs of the future limbs can be seen with a microscope when the embryo is only ten days old. By the end of the sixth week, however, although the embryo is only about 2.5 centimetres long, the tiny limbs are visible to the naked eye. The fact that the arm buds develop slightly earlier than do those for the legs was thought to account for the greater frequency of arm damage, in thalidomide victims, with the radius or ulna (the forearm bones), or both, being absent or defective. In extreme cases, the humerus (or upper arm bone) also failed to appear. The worst cases had neither arms nor legs, rendering them highly vulnerable to pneumonia because of their inability to turn over in their cots or to take unassisted exercise.

There were other effects, too, including hemangioma (or strawberry mark), saddle-shaped or flattened noses, missing external ears and internal auditory canals situated unusually low in the head, paralysis of one side of the face, and malformations of the internal organs involving the alimentary tract and the circulatory system. Most of the affected children turned out to be of normal intelligence.

The first angle of attack adopted by those looking for the cause was to check for any hereditary problems. One team based in Münster had soon completed a study of thirty-four cases and found that there appeared to be no hereditary contribution to these victims of the thalidomide syndrome, or phocomelia as the doctors called it. The inevitable conclusion was that some unknown environmental agent was affecting the embryo at some point between the third and sixth week of pregnancy, a period when most women are ignorant of the fact that they are actually pregnant.

The next question was whether the agent might be a virus, given that infection by rubella, or German measles, can result in severe deformities. In the rubella 'epidemic' in Britain during

1978–9, a hundred babies were born with congenital abnormalities associated with their mothers having contracted the
disease. But rubella had not previously resulted in phocomelia,
better known as the 'seal limb' syndrome. Even more suspicious
was the fact that the outbreak of cases had not begun abruptly.

Fig 4·8   **Fig 4·9**   **Fig 4·10**

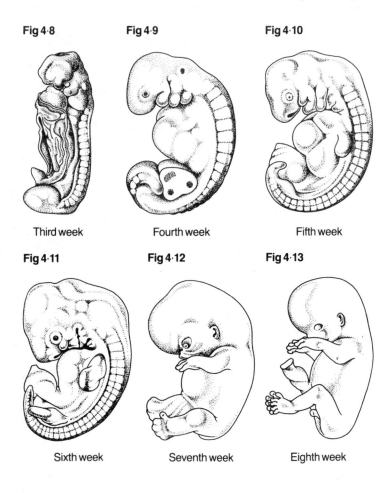

Third week   Fourth week   Fifth week

Fig 4·11   **Fig 4·12**   **Fig 4·13**

Sixth week   Seventh week   Eighth week

Figure 4.8–4.13 The key period in the development of the human
embryo, at least as far as the teratogen thalidomide was concerned, ran
from the third week after conception through the eighth week. The effects
appeared when the mother took the drug during the fourth, fifth or sixth
week of pregnancy – a period when the limbs, ears, intestines, heart and
blood vessels are forming and going through the early stages of growth.
(*Source*: Thaussig, *Scientific American*, August 1962, pp. 29–35)

Instead, it was increasing fairly steadily, and was confined, at that stage, to West Germany. By the time paediatricians gathered for a meeting in Düsseldorf at the end of 1961 some of them were also speculating that the cause of the problem might be fallout from nuclear bomb testing.

But two investigators, Dr William McBride (an obstetrician based in Sydney, Australia) and Professor Widukind Lenz (head of the children's clinic at Hamburg University, West Germany), had independently come to the correct conclusion. Dr McBride had delivered a number of children suffering from the syndrome and had pinpointed Distival as the common factor. Professor Lenz, on the other hand, had been sending out lengthy questionnaires to the parents of deformed children, asking about any exposure to X-rays, drugs, hormones, detergents, foods and food preservatives, contraceptive measures and pregnancy tests. In his early returns he noticed that about 20 per cent of the mothers were reporting having taken Contergan during pregnancy.

On 8 November 1961 it occurred to him that Contergan could be the culprit. He promptly contacted his sample again and asked specifically about Contergan – and 50 per cent reported having

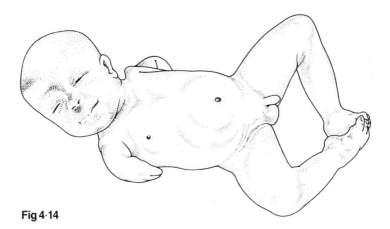

Fig 4·14

Figure 4.14   Thalidomide victims typically suffer from deformed arms and hands, with other deformities affecting the legs and feet, the ears, digestive tract, heart and large blood vessels. The infant shown above also has hemangioma, or strawberry mark, which is harmless, on his forehead, nose and upper lip. The intelligence of most of these children was not affected by thalidomide. (*Source*: as for Figures 4.8–4.13)

used the drug. Many of those now reporting having used it commented that they had considered the drug too innocuous to mention on the earlier questionnaire. The manufacturers were still struggling to save a drug that Grünenthal had called the 'apple of our eye'. But even the sceptics were soon persuaded, and on 26 November the company withdrew the drug. One obstetrician in West Germany was among those who promptly began to ask women who were still pregnant whether they had used Contergan. He checked with sixty-five women, of whom only one had taken Contergan. He declared that if she had an abnormal baby, he would believe Lenz. Unhappily, she did.

The investigators hit a number of snags in trying to pin down the specific details of exposure and effect. In Hamburg, for example, Professor Lenz had decided to check the exact connection between phocomelia and Contergan, intending to identify reliably the date or dates of exposure. He set fairly rigorous standards in his research, considering the use of Contergan proven only if he had in front of him a photocopy of a prescription or hospital record, a requirement which was particularly difficult given that Contergan had been sold over the counter, without a prescription, before April 1961. The various other countries which were beginning to be affected had at least insisted on prescriptions.

Another problem was that nurses in West German hospitals, in the words of Professor Taussig, 'dispensed sleeping tablets as freely as nurses in the US give laxatives'. When she visited West Germany shortly after the first cases were confirmed, Professor Lenz told her of one case which illustrated the nature of the problem. 'The attending physician swore that the mother had not received Contergan,' Lenz told her, 'although her baby had been born with phocomelia. The physician insisted that he had prescribed a different sedative. At the pharmacy Lenz found the prescription marked by the druggist: "Drug not in stock. Contergan given instead".'

By the end of 1961, at least 5,000 cases of children suffering from phocomelia had been reported, yet one of the world's largest markets had escaped almost unscathed. Dr Kelsey's experience with the use of quinine against malaria during the Second World War had, in her own words, made her 'particularly conscious of the fact that the fetus or newborn may be, pharmacologically, an entirely different organism from the adult'. Before Merrell, the company wishing to market thalidomide in the USA, had had time to complete the test programme which would have answered her questions, the outbreaks of phocomelia in West Germany and elsewhere had scuttled the drug's chances. Only a few cases emerged in the USA, such as the West German wife of an American serviceman who returned to the States with Contergan in her luggage – and later gave birth to twins suffering from phocomelia.

One of the more remarkable features of the thalidomide story was that, while many people who took the drug suffered from neurological side-effects, many of the mothers who gave birth to deformed children showed no effects at all. The lesson, and this was confirmed by experience in the aftermath of the Minamata Bay disaster, was that the embryo or foetus may be dramatically affected by a teratogen with no signs of maternal toxicity at all.

While some companies had carried out some research on the possible reproductive effects of some products prior to the thalidomide scandal, there can be no question that thalidomide and its effects on human reproduction gave teratology, the study of birth defects, an enormous boost. By 1969, the US Panel on the Teratogenicity of Pesticides, part of the Mrak Commission, recommended that all of the pesticides then in use 'be tested for teratogenicity in the near future in two or more mammalian species chosen on the basis of the closest metabolic and pharmacologic similarity to human beings possible'. Indeed, an increasingly broad spectrum of pharmaceuticals and chemicals have since been subjected to such tests, many of which will be discussed in later chapters.

This increasing research effort soon began to uncover a number of important facts about the behaviour of the foetal system when exposed to teratogens or other chemical threats, and about the ways in which these substances can move across the placental barrier. It emerged, for example, that the chance of a compound crossing the placental barrier falls with increasing molecular weight, increasing electrical charge, and decreasing lipid solubility. In other words, a compound which has a low molecular weight, a low electrical charge and a high lipid solubility ought to be the object of considerable suspicion.

Some such compounds can penetrate the placenta by means of simple diffusion, while others manage to do so by means of active transport (the transfer of a substance, especially through a cell membrane, from areas where its concentration is high to areas

where it is low) and by means of pinocytosis (involving the ingestion of surrounding fluid by a cell, typically involving local
invagination of a membrane and the entrapment of a minute drop
of fluid in the cytoplasm, as a vesicle). Not surprisingly, given the
placenta's complex and vigorous metabolism, some problem
materials may be the subject of biotransformation in the placenta
– which could conceivably result in an even more powerful
teratogen.

The foetus, however, may also be protected from such substances by the mother, often via detoxification of the substance in
the mother's liver (with the proviso that some break-down
products, or metabolites, may prove even more toxic), excretion by
the kidneys or in the bile, or via the binding of the substance to
plasma proteins which make it impossible for it to cross the
placenta. The foetus may also be protected by the mother's unwitting storage of the chemical threat about her person. In the case
of DDT and other lipid-soluble compounds, for example, the
mother's fatty tissue acts as a reservoir, reducing the amount of
the compound circulating in her bloodstream. Similarly, some
heavy metals are deposited in the mother's bones. Indeed, it may
well be the case that variations in this ability to 'bank' problem
chemicals in various parts of the body accounts for the different
levels of susceptibility seen in different species of animal.

These variations between species are partly responsible for the
difficulties facing those whose business it is to test chemicals on
animals before they are used by people. The final test animal is
always the man, woman or child who takes the drug or is exposed
to the suspect chemical. The more of us who take the drug or are
exposed to the chemical, the more likely it is that some unsuspected
side-effect will emerge, partly because of the genetic factors involved. A prime example of this problem was Debendox.

When its manufacturer was forced to withdraw the drug in
1983, Debendox had been in use for well over twenty years. In
Britain alone, where it had been granted a product licence in 1972
and was available without a prescription until 1978, an estimated
four million British women had taken the drug and about 100,000
prescriptions were being issued each year. Worldwide, an estimated thirty-three million women had used the drug during pregnancy, to provide relief from the symptoms of 'morning sickness',
involving nausea and vomiting. The company involved was the
same company which had tried to introduce thalidomide into the

US market, Merrell, although by the time that Debendox was withdrawn Merrell had sold its pharmaceutical division to Dow.

Debendox, in fact, was the third Merrell drug to come under scrutiny because of side-effects. In the early 1960s the company, one of the longest-established and largest in its field, was forced to withdraw Triparonao, an anti-cholesterol drug, because it was responsible for hair loss and, even more seriously, for the formation of cataracts leading to blindness in some patients. Merrell was indicted by a grand jury on counts of knowingly making false, fictitious and fraudulent statements to the relevant control authorities, and was fined $80,000. Nearly 300 civil lawsuits followed in the wake of that indictment, at a cost to the company running into hundreds of millions of dollars. The second catastrophe, as far as Merrell was concerned, was thalidomide, which it had marketed in Canada and distributed widely for clinical trials in the United States.

When it came to Debendox, however, Merrell-Dow Pharmaceuticals decided that it was not going to go quietly to the slaughter. 'Regulatory and health agencies around the world and the overwhelming majority of independent experts agree that the available evidence does not demonstrate an association between the use of Debendox and birth defects,' it declared, although it admitted that no amount of support for the drug would overcome 'the continuing ill-informed opinion and attack coming from outside the proper medical and scientific arena'. Or, as the company's president, David Sharrock, put it, 'Bendectin [the trade name for Debendox in the United States] is safe and effective. We are taking this action for economic reasons. The real losers are the women of the future.'

However, by the time the company stopped production of Debendox, the drug was the subject of over 250 court cases in the United States, the central allegation being that it caused birth defects when taken during early pregnancy – with the alleged side-effects including deformed limbs, missing fingers, and heart and stomach defects. The company's decision came just thirteen days after a US jury awarded $750,000 (£468,000) to the family of twelve-year-old Mary Oxendine, who had been born with a shortened right hand and missing fingers after her mother took the drug during pregnancy. In an earlier law-suit, initiated in 1980 by Mrs Betty Mekdeci on behalf of her son David, the award had been a mere $20,000, compared to the $12 million the plaintiffs sought. The Oxendine ruling put new heart into those with outstanding suits.

On 14 July 1984, Dow Chemical agreed, in an out-of-court settlement, to pay $120 million to 700 Americans who had claimed that Bendectin had caused birth defects in their children. The company insisted that the agreement 'should not be construed as an admission of liability'. The 400 British families which were also hoping for compensation recognized that they would have a difficult time of it: UK law requires the plaintiff to prove that the drug was capable of causing birth defects.

Whichever way one looked at it, however, Debendox could not have been a particularly strong teratogen if thirty-three million women and their children escaped unscathed, unlike diethylstilbestrol (DES), a drug prescribed between 1940 and 1970 to prevent miscarriages. It was found that male foetuses exposed to DES suffered from a higher incidence of sperm abnormalities, undescended testes, hypospadias and epididymal cysts. Female foetuses were affected even worse: they suffered not only from teratogenic effects, but also from cancers which developed in later life. The birth defects centred around the genitalia, with the females having such problems as cervical and vaginal adenosis, hypoplastic cervixes and uterine anomalies. Later in life, they showed a higher incidence of premature deliveries when pregnant. DES also had the unhappy distinction of being the only known transplacental carcinogen in humans, causing vaginal clear-cell adenocarcinoma in some female foetuses exposed to it in the womb.

Unusually, the effects of DES seemed to be independent of the dose received, a fact which was particularly worrying in light of the fact that an estimated fifty million people had been exposed to trace amounts of DES after it was used as a growth promoter in beef cattle and poultry. And, just in case this all sounds like an historical problem, it is worth pointing out that there are those who strongly suspect that DES is still being used as a growth promoter in some countries, and who worry that a market could well develop even in those countries where it has been banned. In Puerto Rico, for example, paediatric endocrinologist Dr Carmen Sáenz was one of the scientists who, in 1983, attributed the fact that over 3,000 cases of premature puberty had been reported to the use of DES or similar growth promoters. Girls of only five or six had begun to develop breasts and had started menstruating, while some of the young boys who had been affected had started to develop such feminine features as breast tissue. By using a private detective, Dr Sáenz showed that DES could be bought across the counter at agricultural merchants on the island, despite the fact that it was banned in Puerto Rico. She concluded that artificially fattened chickens could well be the source of the problem, since children who switched to other foods tended to lose their symptoms.

These charges triggered a series of government investigations and a temporary drop of 30 per cent in chicken sales. Puerto Rico's meat and milk industries responded by arguing that the whole thing was a plot by food importers to sabotage local production. Many companies took full-page advertisements in the local newspapers defending their products. And, to be fair, there were other suspects.

The condition of accelerated puberty is known as premature thelarche, and there had been previous outbreaks both in the Middle East and in Italy. In the Middle East, the problem was eventually attributed to milk from a cow that had been receiving DES injections. But diet is not the only possible cause of the condition. Insecticides such as DDT have been found to cause the disorder, as has the manufacture of oestrogen-based birth control pills. In one case reported in Poland during 1967, it was found that parents working in a birth control pill factory had been inadvertently exposing their children to oestrogen powder which they had brought home on their working clothes. But the Centers for Disease Control in Atlanta were unable initially to uncover any link between the problem in Puerto Rico and the island's birth control pill factories which produce some 90 per cent of the US supply.

Before turning to look at the teratogenic effects of some heavy metals and pesticides as examples of environmental teratogens, it is worth just commenting on a number of threats to the foetus which are so commonplace that they tend to be ignored by many mothers. The first of these is smoking. When Dr Richard Kurzel and Dr Curtis Cetrulo of the Tufts University School of Medicine reviewed the literature on the effects of pollutants on human reproduction, they concluded, 'The most serious source of air pollution to a pregnant woman is cigarette smoke, because it exposes the unborn baby to high levels of carbon monoxide, hydrogen cyanide, cadmium, nicotine and polycyclic aromatic compounds such as benzo(a)pyrene, which can cross the placenta.'

Carbon monoxide diffuses across the placenta with relative ease and the carboxyhaemoglobin concentration in the foetus can exceed that in the mother by between 10 and 15 per cent. Experiments with rats have shown that carbon monoxide exposure leads to decreased birth weight and increased perinatal mortality. It is difficult, however, to distinguish between the effects of carbon monoxide in cigarette smoke and those of some of the other constituents. When the Guy's Hospital Medical School team considered carbon monoxide, it concluded that 'where exposure is sufficient to cause unconsciousness in the mother, then there seems to be a high risk that the foetus will die. Lower levels of carbon monoxide exposure may still adversely affect the foetus, producing neurological damage or reduced foetal growth.' No evidence has been found to suggest that carbon monoxide is teratogenic, however, but hydrogen cyanide, also found in cigarette smoke, may inhibit the development of the foetal central nervous system. Researchers at Johns Hopkins University, Baltimore, believe that maternal smoking can damage parts of the foetal brain involved in learning – at least as far as experimental rats are concerned. Professor Neville Butler of the Royal Hospital for Sick Children in Bristol followed up 12,000 children and believes the Johns Hopkins results hold for humans too.

Another commonplace activity with potentially serious implications for the foetus is the drinking of large amounts of coffee during pregnancy, largely because of the resulting intake of caffeine. Caffeine is added to soft drinks, to chocolate and to analgesics, but is a natural constituent of coffee and tea. In September 1980 the US Food and Drug Administration warned pregnant women to stop or cut their intake of caffeine because of its potential teratogenicity. Caffeine crosses the human placenta and has been shown to be taken up by the blastocyst, although no evidence exists yet to show conclusively that caffeine is a human teratogen.

When caffeine was tested on rats, with the animals being given the equivalent of between twelve and twenty-four cups of coffee a day, some newborn rats had missing digits, delayed skeletal development and showed growth retardation. One study of 202 cases of human birth defects found a statistically significant higher consumption of coffee in the group of mothers with defective babies. The study, which was controlled for the effects of age and for cigarette and drug consumption, showed an increase in the frequency of birth defects in heavy coffee drinkers, defined as drinking over seven cups a day.

But of all the classes of chemical compounds studied for such effects to date, probably the most significant embryotoxins and teratogens have shown up among organic pesticides and among the metals and their associated compounds. The results of tests on a range of animal species show that a considerable number of metals show teratogenic effects, with mercury and lead included in any listing of metals which are definitely embryotoxic or tera- togenic, and with arsenic, copper, lithium and selenium also coming under suspicion.

As we saw in Chapter 1, inorganic mercury compounds used as catalysts in a plastics plant were released in Minamata Bay, Japan, with some of the metallic and inorganic salts possibly being con- verted to alkyl (including methyl) mercury compounds by anaero- bic bacteria living in the Bay itself. The bulk of the alkyl mercury, however, was discharged from the plant directly, entering the food chain and, by means of bioconcentration, reached unusually high levels in the flesh of the fish caught and eaten in the area.

Variations between the proportions of mothers and children affected underscored the particular susceptibility of the foetus to mercury poisoning. In a study of one group of mothers it was found that in seventeen cases where the child had developed cerebral palsy the mother had experienced no warning symptoms, just a few reporting a numbing of their fingers or fatigue – itself not an uncommon state among pregnant mothers. Among the foetal and post-natal effects recorded were brain damage, manifested as mental retardation, spasticity, chronic seizures and blindness. In one follow-up study of the surviving children in one particular area, it was found that 6 per cent had developed cerebral palsy.

Methyl mercury turned out to have a particular affinity for the foetal nervous system, the dosage being found to accumulate over time and the foetus being shown to trap the mercury selectively. Indeed, the concentration of mercury in the foetal brain turns out to be four times higher than that in the mother's brain, while the level in the foetal blood is about 28 per cent higher than in the mother's blood.

Lead is another problem metal, proving to be embryotoxic and teratogenic in humans, although with milder effects than are found with methyl mercury. The ability of lead to induce abortions has been recognized for a long time and was illegally exploited around the turn of the century to terminate unwanted preg- nancies. The resulting abortion rate was apparently high, but the toll was also high among the mothers treated in this way, with the side-effects including brain damage and blindness. Unlike mercury, however, lead does not appear to be preferentially concentrated in the foetus. It crosses the placenta only if given in high concentrations, tending to concentrate in the foetal bone and liver. It also accumulates in the placenta itself, which may account for its impact on the spontaneous abortion rate.

It is believed that lead's embryotoxicity and teratogenicity are related to its effect on some of the metallo-enzymes which are involved in the process of embryonic differentiation, the process during which a cluster of totipotential cells (cells which can develop into any sort of cell in the mature organism) begin to evolve into distinct organs. It has also been shown to interact with other metals when used in animal experiments, with the introduction of cadmium during experiments on lead toxicity increasing the rate of lead-induced malformations in hamsters – and introducing new malformations.

While cadmium causes the disease in humans now known as 'Itai, Itai', a term used to express agony in Japanese, it has not been shown to have embryotoxic or teratogenic effects in humans. It does cross the placenta and is retained mainly in the foetal liver and kidneys, where it has been shown to accumulate. It is embryotoxic in mice and teratogenic in rats, in which it has been found to cause slow growth, hypoplastic lungs, clubbed feet and cleft palates. In hamsters, cadmium causes craniofacial, brain, eye and limb defects.

Arsenic, whose compounds were used in the past to treat syphilis, is thought unlikely to be a teratogen in humans, although in rats, ewes and hamsters it has been found to cause cleft palates, exencephaly, anophthalmia, microphthalmia and renal agensis. In humans, though, organic arsenicals appear not to cross the placenta, instead accumulating there. Arsenic can be toxic to the human foetus, although the effects can be reduced by administering selenium, which is thought to compete with arsenic for sites where the damage is caused. Selenium, however, is toxic to embryos and teratogenic in its own right, according to tests in hens, sheep and calves. One reported side-effect involved shortened limbs.

Any product containing any of these metals is now clearly a prime candidate for teratogenicity testing, although one law quoted by teratologists suggests that any compound can be teratogenic if given to the right species, at the right dose and at the right time. That said, however, the testing of many products for human teratogenicity has tended to occur in highly uncontrolled situations. Reliable, well-documented studies of the teratogenic effects of such products as pesticides are conspicuous by their absence. Only the organomercurials are conclusively known to be human teratogens.

Reproductive failure in wildlife because of exposure to pesticides was one of the central themes in Rachel Carson's *Silent Spring*, and the evidence has continued to support her conclusions. To take just one example, it has been reported that California sea-lions which delivered their pups prematurely were later found to have in their fat levels of chlorinated pesticides, including DDT, DDD and DDE, which were eight times higher than those found in sea-lions which had been able to deliver their pups normally. The premature pups were themselves found to have twice as much of these compounds in their fat as the normal pups.

Clearly, because of their lipid solubility and their persistence, the organochlorine pesticides are obvious suspects as far as foetal contamination is concerned – and there is certainly no doubt that they can cross the placenta. In one study reported in 1969, DDT, DDE, lindane, dieldrin and heptachlorepoxide were found in the foetal blood contained in the umbilical cords of ten stillborn infants, with the levels approximating those found in adults. Japanese researchers have also attributed some foetal deaths and malformations to the spraying of field workers with organophosphorous insecticides. Another study which underscored the difficulties often experienced in interpreting the available evidence focused on the levels of DDE in the blood of premature and non-premature infants, and found that the premature infants had between three and four times as much DDE in their tissues as did the control group of infants born normally. The question remained whether this accurately reflected elevated exposure of the premature infants to DDE or whether, instead, it reflected the fact that the premature infants may have had less body fat in which to store typical levels of DDE.

One extremely potent foetotoxicant and teratogen, however, is 2,3,7,8-tetrachlorodibenzo-*p*-dioxin (TCDD), which is a contaminant formed from chlorophenols during the manufacture of herbicides such as 2,4-D and 2,4,5-T. These came under suspicion during the Vietnam war when 'Agent Orange' was used in the

American defoliation programme and have since been the subject of considerable controversy.

A class of pesticides known as the phthalimides are also under suspicion because of their structural similarity to thalidomide, although no birth defects have been documented in mammals. Defects did show up in chicks, however, and captan, folpet and difolatan are known to be mutagenic in bacteria – while captan has an alkylating capability, a characteristic of some problem chemicals.

With such a large number of chemicals now known to be actual or (more commonly) potential foetotoxins or teratogens, it is no wonder that a growing number of people are becoming aware of the problem – and are expressing their concern. Communities around the world, whether at Love Canal, Seveso or in the rural areas of Thailand (see p. 231), are realizing that the chemicals which they or others produce, use and dispose of, with varying degrees of care, may affect a whole range of reproductive activities in wildlife, in domestic and farmed animals, and, most worryingly, in themselves and in their children.

Scientists, meanwhile, have been trying to establish what level of birth defects can be accepted as 'normal'. Many factors are involved, including genetic considerations. In some countries cultural factors may aggravate this genetic dimension of the problem. Take Turkey as an example. Turkish geneticists have estimated that at least 10 per cent of the marriages which take place in rural Turkey are between first cousins or between uncles and their nieces. In some parts of the country, including eastern Anatolia, the proportion of such close-kin (or consanguineous) marriages may be as high as 40 per cent. As a result, Turkish doctors encounter fairly considerable numbers of patients whose problems are genetically based. In one village, there are twenty people suffering from hermaphroditism, while in another a dominant gene has been isolated – resulting in the world's largest single community of muscular dystrophy sufferers.

While it may be difficult to distinguish between teratogenic effects caused by such factors and those caused by chemicals or other environmental teratogens, some scientists are beginning to wonder whether there may not be some much more subtle teratogens at work. Dr Tesh of Life Science Research is among these, and one of the reasons why he is worried is that, far from the child's development being complete at birth, some elements of the central nervous system continue to develop for perhaps two years after birth.

'With thalidomide,' he says, 'which produced gross deformities that were immediately recognizable at birth, it took some two years to recognize that any problem existed and a further two or three years to identify the causal agent. If one considers an agent capable of producing more subtle changes,' he continues, thinking in terms of the impairment of learning ability, memory, the power of concentration and of intelligence itself, 'then what would be the chances of identifying such an agent? At birth one would have an apparently normal, healthy infant which would grow and be in junior school, perhaps six to eight years old, before it was realized that any problem existed. Assuming there was an impairment,' he points out, 'trying to trace the causative factor would be extremely difficult and even if it were possible, the number of affected children could be of almost epidemic proportions before the agent responsible was withdrawn.'

Meanwhile, a considerable number of chemicals continue to emerge in animal tests as embryotoxins or teratogens, generally with no conclusive evidence on their effects on humans. Examples of substances now known to be embryotoxic or embryolethal in some animal species (but not in our own species) are chloroform, dichloromethane, ethylene dichloride, ethylene oxide, inorganic mercury, nitrogen dioxide, polybrominated biphenyls, selenium, tetrachloroethylene, thallium, trichloroethylene, vinyl chloride and xylene. Those which have emerged as animal teratogens, but not yet as human teratogens, are arsenic, benzo(a)pyrene, chlordifluoromethane, chloroprene, monomethyl formamide, acrylonitrile, methyl ethyl ketone, tellurium and vinyl chloride. Arsenic, benzo(a)pyrene and vinyl chloride have also been found to act as transplacental carcinogens in some animal species.

Interestingly, in the case of DES, there was a significant breakthrough in the US courts early in 1984 which promised (or threatened, depending on your viewpoint) to remove a key obstacle to the prosecution of manufacturers of products which prove to be carcinogens, teratogens or mutagens. The Michigan Supreme Court ruled that Loretta T. Robu, a woman who contracted a form of cancer linked with the DES her mother had taken during pregnancy, could sue *all* the manufacturers of DES, with the costs allocated according to market share. Previously, plaintiffs had to prove that DES manufactured by one particular company was to blame out of the more than 300 to some extent involved. The implications of the ruling did not escape the lawyers of major corporations likely to be caught in similar cases. They were appalled.

But, while birth defects and cancer are themselves appalling problems, with unthinkable consequences for those individuals, families and communities affected, there is an even more worrying possibility facing our species: that some of the chemicals which we have synthesized, distributed, used and disposed of with relatively little thought for the consequences may prove to be mutagens. A mutagen is an agent which induces inheritable genetic change, an alteration called a mutation. Virtually all mutations represent a handicap, of varying degrees of importance, as far as the survival of the species is concerned.

CHAPTER FIVE

A
MUTANT'S
INHERITANCE

When facts are few and far between, suspicions breed like mice. Sometimes, too, the available facts emerge in a form which leaves them vulnerable to reinterpretation by suspicious minds. One does not need a particularly long memory to recall occasions when widely accepted 'facts' were discredited. Today's facts, at best, are only as good as today's science – and scientists, the more suspicious among us might observe, spend their time proving that what their predecessors took to be facts were no such thing.

'I'm horrified,' said one American mother of two when she heard that a new report on the health effects of the Love Canal toxic waste dump published by the Atlanta-based Centers for Disease Control concluded that there had been 'no increase in abnormalities' among forty-six residents or former residents of the Love Canal area near Niagara Falls. Although she suspected that chemicals seeping up from the dump had caused the birth defects diagnosed in one of her children, the report seemed scientifically sound. It had compared the sample's chromosomes, the threadlike particles of DNA which transmit hereditary characteristics from one genera-tion to the next, with those of a control group of fifty people living about a mile (1.6 kilometres) from the dump.

But who can blame the Love Canal residents for being confused? Another woman, Lois Gibbs, who had spearheaded a campaign to ensure the evacuation of families from the area following an earlier report which suggested that Love Canal residents *had* suffered chromosomal damage, was not alone in insisting that this latest study had been 'released deliberately to confuse and cause a smoke screen around the Canal'.

Whatever the facts of the matter, the public reaction to actual or suspected contamination with such materials as dioxin has much in common with the psychological 'fall-out' which followed the Three Mile Island nuclear accident. And there is another link between these disasters: both chemicals and ionizing radiation have been shown to trigger mutations in the cells of experimental bacteria and animals. Very few of these mutations can be considered to be remotely beneficial and some may be passed from generation to generation.

If there is one thing which is potentially more frightening than a chemical or other agent which can deform your child as it develops in the apparent safety of the womb, it is a chemical or agent which could impose such a deformity on many of your descendants. A mutation transmitted by a recessive gene, of which more later, might do this, while one transmitted in a dominant gene would almost certainly ensure that *all* your descendants suffered.

The most insidious and worrying aspect of carcinogens is that they can involve a time-lag of decades between exposure and the emergence of the resulting cancer. With mutation-causing agents, or mutagens, and where germ cells (eggs or sperm) are concerned, this time-lag would stretch into generations. Mutagens, in short, can increase the mutation rate either in germ cells, which may cause an increase of genetic disease in future generations, or in somatic cells (that is, cells other than germ cells). Mutations in somatic cells are linked with increased incidences of certain cancers in those animals or people exposed to particular mutagens or to mixes of mutagens.

Indeed, any attempt to assess the risks imposed by an increased mutation rate is quite different in kind from most risk-benefit analyses carried out today. When the Committee on Chemical Environmental Mutagens (part of the US National Research Council's Board on Toxicology and Environmental Health Hazards) reported the findings of its study on the genetic impact of chemical mutagens in 1983, it pointed out that 'it is not unusual for the benefits and risks to go to different persons; ideally, there is some form of compensation. However, it is unusual for the benefits and risks to be many generations apart. In the case of chemical mutagens,' it stressed, 'most of the beneficiaries are living now, whereas most of those at risk have not yet been born and perhaps will not be born for many centuries.'

The problem is simply an extreme form of a question which underlies most of today's environmental problems: can we justify carrying out a particular activity, such as clearing tropical rainforests or building up stocks of spent fuels and highly irradiated materials from nuclear power stations and nuclear weapons facilities, knowing that future generations will have to pick up the tab?

'How can our generation objectively weigh benefits to itself against risks to future generations?' the Committee asked. 'In only a few instances – such as soil and water conservation, the preservation of native vegetation and wilderness areas, and the treatment of endangered species – do we give much thought to future generations.' And even then, it is fair to say, future generations often tend to get remarkably short shrift.

The Committee's report attempted to show the other side of the chemical coin, too. 'Each generation,' it cautioned, 'hands benefits to its descendants. We profit by the scientific and technological advances made by our forefathers and the higher living and health standards that we enjoy are parts of this benefit. To the extent that a beneficial chemical increases the knowledge, technology and wealth that our generation passes to the future, we can say that we are offsetting mutagenic effects. That is not intended to argue against all efforts to protect the genetic health of our descendants, but it does argue against a policy so overprotective as to stultify the development of chemicals that benefit us and may benefit future generations as well.'

A wise qualification, for even if we include only possible somatic cell mutations in the equation, leaving aside mutations which might be passed on to future generations, the evidence we shall now review suggests strongly that twentieth-century chemistry has added significantly to the number of mutagens or possible mutagens. Take thalidomide, for example. We have seen how the drug produced an epidemic of birth defects in the early 1960s and the natural assumption would be that it had been totally suspended for use in humans. Not so. At the time of writing as many as a million patients are being treated with thalidomide. They suffer from leprosy and are being treated with the drug on the assumption, now open to question, that it is toxic only to the unborn.

The drug was taken off the market in 1962, and most of the research on its effects was run down or dropped as it became increasingly difficult to track down supplies. But after thalidomide was banned in Europe some stocks were shipped elsewhere, and in Israel a surprise finding gave it a new lease of life. When used to calm a manic leprosy patient, it was also found to play a useful role in controlling the painful lepra reaction of the disease. No one knew why this was happening, just as they still had no idea about the precise mechanisms involved in the production of birth defects. But the results were so promising that thalidomide was increasingly prescribed for non-pregnant leprosy victims.

Later research raises the possibility that the drug may have caused birth defects by triggering gene mutations. If this suspicion proves to be well-founded, hundreds of thousands of patients who have been treated with the drug may be subject to an increased risk of toxic side-effects, including cancer.

The research was carried out in 1973 by Berndt Hagström of Kabi, the Swedish chemical company, which tried for seven years to develop a non-toxic form of thalidomide for use as a sedative. Ultimately, this work proved a dead end, but in the meantime the research results had been suppressed in the interests of commercial secrecy. Hagström used the ubiquitous Ames test, which assesses the ability of a chemical to induce mutations in the genes of bacteria. These tests showed that thalidomide could act as a mutagen.

Hagström reported observing chromosome damage within three hours of feeding thalidomide to mice. Later, in work done outside Kabi, he also found that the embryos of fish and of sea urchins showed severe skeletal damage after the exposure of eggs or sperm to thalidomide. Since sperm consist mainly of genes, the implication was that the observed effects were caused by damaged genes. As we have seen, however, it is almost always possible to find dissenting views. Such is the nature of science. As far as the mutagenic potential of thalidomide is concerned, the opposing views come from scientists at Johns Hopkins University, who have reported finding no mutagenic effects after spending two years subjecting thalidomide to the Ames test. One member of this research group, David Blake, confessed he was surprised that the drug was not showing up as a mutagen, given its known toxicity. Blake commented that a possible explanation could be that the two laboratories had been using different bacterial types in their tests, although it was not possible to resolve the issue unless Kabi published its results.

In fact, an astonishing variety of tests have been devised to test chemicals for possible mutagenicity. The Committee on Chemical Environmental Mutagens, whose work was funded by the US Environmental Protection Agency via the National Academy of Sciences, discussed about fifty in some detail. These used a considerable range of methods and living systems, including bacteria, fungi, mammalian cell cultures and insects. With a growing number of laboratories using a growing number of mutagenicity tests around the world, it is perhaps not surprising that the data base on chemical mutagens has literally exploded.

By the early 1980s, the files of the Environmental Mutagen Information Center in Oak Ridge, Tennessee, contained more than 40,000 publications covering the genetic effects of at least 13,000 different chemicals – and this high figure represents only about a quarter of the total number of chemicals which are thought to be commercially available in the United States.

The study of chemical mutagenicity is of relatively recent origin. The first real evidence suggesting that environmental agents could influence the mutation rate came in the 1920s, when scientists working with fruit-flies and barley showed that X-rays are mutagenic. Then, during the Second World War, classic work by Charlotte Auerbach demonstrated that chemical mutagenesis was a fact of life. Her experiments showed that mustard gas could produce mutations in fruit-flies. Like mustard gas, the first chemical mutagens to be discovered were all highly toxic materials, a fact which led most investigators to assume that non-accidental exposure would be very unlikely. But later research, which showed that seemingly harmless, non-toxic substances could also be highly mutagenic, turned these assumptions on their head.

'Humans have been exposed, inadvertently or deliberately, to mutagens since at least the end of World War II,' says Donald Clive of Burroughs Wellcome's genetic toxicology laboratory, 'and most probably since we arose as a species. With advancing technology came an ever-expanding list of laboratory mutagens: naturally occurring chemical mutagens, such as those which occur in bracken fern, became supplemented by amino acid pyrolysates with the onset of the cooking revolution some time in the Pleistocene epoch; other revolutions followed, including today's industrial and scientific revolutions. The result of some of these factors is a logically deduced, well-intentioned concern over genetic stewardship – protecting the integrity of that meter of information that makes us what we are, and which threads its way from our earliest beginnings a million or so years ago into the unseen future.'

The scientist who achieved the first indisputable demonstration of the mutagenicity of X-rays in fruit-flies, or *Drosophila*, warned of the risk to future generations if germ cells were exposed to ionizing radiation. His words went unheeded for some time, with the early radiation exposure standards being designed simply to protect those exposed from health effects, rather than to protect their germ cells and future generations. The above-ground A-bomb and H-bomb tests of the 1940s and 1950s, with the ensuing radioactive fallout, did a great deal to promote serious consideration of the reproductive effects of radiation, from whatever source.

The research carried out during the Second World War using mustard gas resulted from the observation that injuries from gas weapons sometimes resembled X-ray burns. By the late 1940s, independent reports were beginning to emerge suggesting that other chemicals could act as mutagens, inducing gene and chromosome mutations. As the scientific literature on muta-genesis began to expand, there was some discussion of the possibility that chemical mutagens might constitute a genetic hazard at least as great as radiation, but the threat of imminent nuclear war and the successive nuclear bomb test programmes meant that radiation effects got headline billing. It is worth looking at some of these effects in detail before turning to chemical mutagens.

If your body was exposed to a very high dose of radiation, you could die within weeks. The amount of radiation a body absorbs is expressed in terms of a unit called the *gray*, whose symbol is Gy. It measures the quantity of energy imparted by ionizing radiation to a unit of matter such as tissue. A Gy corresponds to a joule per kilogram. An instantaneous absorbed dose of 5 Gy or more to the whole body would probably be lethal. If, instead, a small area of the body is briefly exposed to a very high dose of radiation, death may not result but there will be other effects. An instantaneous absorbed dose of 5 Gy to an area of the skin would probably cause reddening after a week or so, while a similar dose delivered to the testes or ovaries could cause sterility. If the same total dose were to be delivered over a longer period, there might be no apparent symptoms, but damage may have been inflicted which could produce significant health problems either in the irradiated individual or, if germ cells have been affected or a foetus irradiated in the womb, in that individual's descendants.

If an embryo is exposed to radiation, developmental defects such as a reduction in the diameter of the head might be expected, for this is the period when the child's organs are being formed. If the exposure takes place later in pregnancy, there will be an enhanced risk of cancer in childhood. Consequently, there are typically special restrictions on the radiation doses that fertile or pregnant women can receive if they are employed as radiation workers.

Cancer is the most important 'late effect' of radiation, although the fundamental processes by which cancer is induced in those exposed are not yet fully understood. Whatever these processes may be, however, a greater incidence of various malignancies (or cancers) has been observed in groups of people exposed to radiation at some time in the past. Provided the dose is not overwhelming, we might expect only a relatively small number of those exposed to actually die of cancer, although everyone who has been exposed can be said to have a *probability* of contracting cancer which depends largely on the dose actually received.

If the number of people in an irradiated group is known, and the number of doses they received is recorded accurately, then the number of cancers eventually observed in that group can help in producing what is called a 'risk factor'. If the number of cancers actually observed exceeds the number expected in a similar (but non-irradiated) group, then the excess number of cancers can be attributed to radiation – and the risk factor calculated in terms of the risk of cancer per unit of radiation exposure. To take an example, if a group of 50,000 people had each received a dose of about 2 sieverts (explained below) to a particular organ, say the liver, and if 100 more cases of liver cancer appeared in this group than in the control group, then the risk factor would be 100 divided by 50,000 × 2, or 1 in 1,000 per sievert (10^{-3} Sv^{-1} if you are scientifically minded). The sievert (symbol Sv) measures the 'dose equivalent', or the absorbed radiation dose multiplied by a factor which takes account of the way a particular radiation distributes energy in tissue – which, in turn, influences its capacity for causing harm. For gamma-rays, X-rays and beta particles, the factor is set at 1, whereas for alpha particles the factor is 20. The dose equivalent, which was formerly expressed in a unit called the *rem*, provides an index of risk of harm from exposure of a particular tissue to different forms of radiation. One Sv of alpha radiation to the lung, for instance, is deemed to create the same risk of fatal lung cancer as one Sv of beta radiation.

In the case of the foetus exposed to radiation in the womb, the risk of childhood cancer is calculated to be about 1 in 40 per Sv (or 2.3×10^{-2} Sv^{-1}), which is about twice the overall risk of cancer for the average individual. Risk factors have also been worked out for such irradiated groups as the survivors of the atomic bomb attacks on Hiroshima and Nagasaki, work which is backed up by studies of patients exposed to radiation as part of therapy for non-malignant conditions or for diagnostic purposes, people exposed to intense nuclear fallout during the bomb tests, uranium industry workers and workers in the luminizing industry. Information on these risk factors is reviewed regularly by the United Nations Scientific Committee on the Effects of Atomic Radiation (UNSCEAR), which was set up in 1955.

Apart from cancer, the other important late effect of radiation is hereditary damage, the probability (but not severity) of which depends on the dose. The damage arises through irradiation of the gonads, which produce the sperm cells in males and egg cells in females. Surprisingly, there is no direct evidence of hereditary defects in human offspring which are directly attributable either to natural or to man-made radiation. Even more surprisingly, studies of 71,000 children of survivors of the atomic bombings of Hiroshima and Nagasaki have failed to produce clear evidence of any increases in the incidence of congenital malformations, cyto-genetic abnormalities or in perinatal and childhood mortality rates. It is fair to say, however, that some investigators, such as George R. Hoffman (project director of the US Committee on Chemical Environmental Mutagens study until 1981), see this as evidence of the insensitivity of current population monitoring methods.

Combining the Japanese findings with evidence gleaned from extensive studies on the hereditary damage induced in experi-mental animals, mainly mice, exposed to ionizing radiation, UNSCEAR has calculated a risk factor for serious hereditary damage to humans: its value is about 1 in 50 Sv (2×10^{-2} Sv^{-1}), when all later generations are taken into account. About half of this damage would be expressed in the children and grandchildren of the irradiated individuals, suggesting a risk factor of 1 in 100 per Sv.

*

All this work on radiation effects has contributed enormously to our understanding of mutagenesis in general. 'The growth of the chemical aspects of mutagenesis and its correlation with carcino-genesis has been so great,' concluded the UK Committee on Mutagenicity of Chemicals in Food, Consumer Products and the Environment (CMCFCPE) in 1981, 'that the literature is now much more extensive than that on radiation mutagenesis, yet it must not be forgotten that it is the fundamental knowledge gained from radiation studies that underlies our understanding of the way chemicals can act and in turn gives strong support to our realiza-tion of the potential dangers of chemical mutagens.' The Com-mittee pointed out that 'no single chemical possesses a mutagenic data base that remotely approaches that available for X-rays'.

To date, several thousand chemicals have proved mutagenic in at least one of the commonly used test systems. These chemicals include some which, like food additives and hair dyes, have been in common usage. Over a hundred chemicals which are known to cause cancer in experimental animals have also proved to act as mutagens, including at least twenty chemicals which are known human carcinogens. However, as the CMCFCPE stressed, 'sub-stances do not always fall conveniently into two categories: mutagen and non-mutagen. The mutagenicity of some substances can be detected with ease, and of other substances only with difficulty.'

The problem is that, in direct contrast to the belief, widespread until the 1960s, that most mutagenic chemicals acted in the cell in exactly the same form as they entered the body, many mutagens are activated by the body biochemistry of those exposed to them. Of course, it was known that some of the body's enzymes were able to convert chemicals into other substances, but it was thought that this generally involved the inactivation or detoxification of such drugs and chemicals. Some chemicals have proved muta-genic in their original form, but we now know that many are not active until they are metabolized, and, it transpires, toxi-fication and detoxification often run in tandem within the same cell, with the various enzymes involved being controlled by genes.

As the Committee on Chemical Environmental Mutagens con-cluded, 'the recognition that many innocuous substances become mutagenic because of activating enzymes in the body has led to an entirely different view of mutagen detection. It is no longer sufficient to assume that a chemical is harmless on the grounds that it is non-mutagenic in a simple (test) system. Many chemicals are not mutagenic themselves, but are converted into mutagens in the body, usually in the liver. Reactions with chemicals of external origin lead to a complicated and delicate balance of toxification and detoxification. Intermediate products are often highly active and can interact with DNA in ways that lead to mutation. It remains unclear why so many harmless chemicals are converted into mutagens, but the fact is not in doubt.' To take just one example, a somatic mutagen such as benzopyrene causes cancer only when it has been converted into epoxides.

Clearly, there are some aspects of chemical mutagenesis which are rather different to what we might expect from our experience with radiation mutagenesis. If, for instance, a particular set of tissues is irradiated in the human body, then all the cells in those tissues are going to be affected; but in chemical mutagenesis there can be no such certainty. To discover whether a particular chemical is likely to act as a mutagen, it is necessary not only to find out whether people can ingest, inhale or otherwise absorb it, but also to find out whether the chemical, or any active metabolites, can reach the germ cells. Sadly, anyone wishing to find out how such chemicals are metabolized in the body will find that pharmacokinetic studies required to track chemicals and metabolites around the body are still in their infancy.

Because of the importance of activation in turning an otherwise innocent chemical into a potential mutagen, chemical test systems need to mimic the metabolism of the human body – which, as we have seen, is in some respects still far from fully understood. However, extracts from rat livers have been found to be effective in mimicking many of the human metabolic processes when added to test systems, with many substances emerging as potential mutagens only when such activating substances are included. Mutation tests are run both with and without such substances, to identify those chemicals which would be mutagenic with no further activation needed and those which need an activation stage (or activation stages) to become mutagenic.

One of the more important findings to surface from such research confirms that different mammals, and even different strains of the same mammal, can vary very significantly indeed in the way in which they metabolize particular chemicals. This makes it very difficult to draw hard and fast conclusions about possible effects in humans from results obtained in, say, experimental rats. Another implication of the genetic control of the enzymes which toxify and detoxify chemicals in the body is that, as the National Academy of Sciences (NAS) study put it, 'people can be expected to differ in their constellations of enzymes, and therefore in their susceptibility to mutagens. Some examples are known, but this field is in its infancy. It would be desirable to take account of the fact that some chemicals that are non-mutagenic for most people may be highly mutagenic for a few. It is not yet possible to gauge this sensitivity, but it is very likely to be an important part of the mutation protection of the future.' (Chapter 8 looks at some of the genetic screening tests which are already being used in the chemical industry and elsewhere in an attempt to identify those who are likely to be particularly susceptible to specific chemicals.)

In welcoming the publication of the NAS report, which it described as 'exceedingly intelligent', the science journal *Nature* commented that 'the ideal, of course, would be that there should be a full understanding of what happens metabolically to particular chemicals in mammalian cells (in germ as well as somatic cells), and such a full catalogue of possible interactions with nuclear DNA that the prediction of mutagenicity would be possible. For the time being, however,' the leader writer warned, 'such an objective is entirely beyond the bounds of what can be attained. So the best hope is that some long-pocketed agency such as the Environmental Protection Agency should support an empirical attempt to discover what there is in common between the chemicals – the list is short – known to be mutagens of the germ-line.'

The advice which the Environmental Protection Agency (EPA) received from the Committee on Chemical Environmental Mutagens, an offshoot of the National Academy of Science's Board on Toxicology and Environmental Health Hazards, was, to use *Nature*'s words, 'surprisingly pragmatic'. It suggested that if the EPA was committed to spotting inheritably mutagenic chemicals before they cause damage, its best course would be to rely on a combination of tests – including a version of the Ames test and an assay of a chemical's potential for causing chromosome breaks in cultured mammalian cells (such as those derived from hamster tissues).

The NAS report was unusual, however, in not going overboard in favour of more legislation. *Nature* was not alone in supporting this decision, but its reaction nicely summarized some of the arguments for and against legislation. 'What trigger-happy lawyers and their paymasters must be made to understand,' it suggested, 'is that the Environmental Protection Agency has asked an interesting question, that the National Academy of Sciences has given an intelligent answer, and that there is, for the time being, no way of telling what should be done to protect people against the hypothetical hazard of germ-line mutations by chemicals except by the support of basic research.'

Of course, one would expect a publication dedicated to the reporting of basic research results to support the call for further research, but if we review our knowledge of mutagenesis to date it becomes only too clear that there remain significant gaps in our understanding of what makes a mutagen a mutagen – and of what stops some apparent mutagens, which have caused chromosome breaks and other genetic damage in such warning systems as the Ames test, from acting as mutagens in people.

In the UK, the CMCFCPE also underscored the gaps in our knowledge, ultimately plumping for a basic test package which, on paper at least, had many similarities to the test package proposed by the NAS. It considered that, 'in the light of present knowledge, the great majority of potentially hazardous chemicals can be detected by a combination of four test procedures designed to probe the hereditary machinery sequentially, at increasing levels of complexity.' This package, which the Committee stressed was basic, involves three *in vitro* tests (carried out in test-tubes, for example) and one *in vivo* test, involving the study of the behaviour of the chemical and its metabolites in live animals. The first of the recommended *in vitro* tests was the Ames test which, the Committee said, 'is incontestably the most widely validated system in the field of genetic toxicology and is believed to be the most sensitive'. However, once the activity of a test chemical has been demonstrated in such a simple bacterial system, the Committee recommended that 'all further testing should be carried out using mammalian systems'.

Let us consider first some of the contributions which the basic science, so keenly promoted by the NAS and by *Nature*, has already made to our understanding of the genetic bedrock of human reproduction. The key to this understanding, clearly, is the revolutionary research which has been carried out since the 1950s in molecular biology, particularly that focusing on the role of de-oxyribonucleic acid (DNA). The key breakthrough here was the discovery by Watson and Crick in 1953 of the 'double helix', the double-stranded helical structure of DNA. Their findings triggered an explosive mushrooming in our knowledge of the molecular basis of heredity which is absolutely fundamental to our understanding of the process of mutagenesis.

The recognition that the DNA molecule is a double helix, which peels apart to produce two separate templates for the assembly of further DNA molecules, helped explain the remarkable accuracy of DNA replication. This accuracy, in turn, depends on the activities of hordes of biochemical repairmen, in the form of enzymes. The striking thing about DNA, as the CMCFCPE put it, is that this basic building-block for living systems is not as robust as one might expect.

'In view of the faithfulness of the transmission of genetic information through the generations,' the Committee noted, 'it is perhaps surprising to learn that DNA is itself not a particularly stable molecule and that it can be damaged relatively easily. The apparent stability of the system derives from the associated complex of proteins and enzymes, which not only subserve the basic functions of DNA (replication and transcription) but also have the capacity to repair various kinds of damage to the base sequence.' This damage can involve either of the spiralling strands which make up the DNA molecule.

A veritable army of enzymes – endonucleases, exonucleases and polymerase – keep the DNA molecule under constant surveillance. If any small chemical defects are spotted on one of the strands, the affected areas are snipped out and replaced, using the other strand as a template. There are also a variety of other repair mechanisms which replace or rebuild damaged sections of the DNA molecule, and the manipulation of these processes has become an important technique in mutation research.

We have mentioned transcription without explaining it. DNA transcription can occur throughout the life of a cell, unlike replication. Simply put, the process of transcription involves the dispatch of a set of blueprints from the DNA strands to the ribosomes, which are effectively protein factories, where they are used to construct polypeptides and then proteins.

The basic unit in talking about genetic material is the gene. Physically, a gene consists of a sequence of points on either of the two spiralling strands of DNA and serves as a blueprint for assembling, say, a polypeptide, or it may contain the information defining some controlling or regulatory gene function. The typical human somatic cell contains forty-six chromosomes, each of which is made up of genes together with their associated protein and enzyme support systems. In the process of cell division, each chromosome replicates itself, so that each of the two 'daughter' cells contains its own complete set of chromosomes. This process, which is called 'mitosis', ensures that, barring errors along the way, each cell in our bodies contains the same number of chromosomes as the fertilized egg (or zygote) from which each of us began.

All higher organisms are made up of an almost infinite variety of cells, with the trillions of cells found in each of our bodies having been produced from that original fertilized egg by way of countless cell divisions. Some investigators have tended to use the term 'genetic effect' to cover any change induced by a mutagen in a cell, be it a somatic or germ cell, because all cells contain DNA, but the only mutations which can affect future generations are those which take place in germ cells – in the sperm and egg which come together to form the zygote from which all else springs.

The business of manufacturing sperm and egg cells, which are collectively known as 'gametes', proceeds along different lines from those which guide mitosis (the process by which a cell nucleus divides into two). In meiosis, two divisions of the cell nucleus are accompanied by only a single division of the chromosomes, so that the resulting gametes have only twenty-three chromosomes each. This halving of the chromosomes is not random: the chromosomes occur in pairs and the gametes get one chromosome from each pair, with fertilization, if it takes place, ensuring that the resulting zygote has the necessary twenty-three pairs of chromosomes. This means that each zygote contains one chromosome from each of its parents' chromosome pairs and meiosis also includes a process called 'crossing over', during which the male and female chromosomes pair up and exchange parts. Clearly, the resulting child is the product of a fairly thorough scrambling of the chromosomes of its mother and father.

Almost all our hereditary traits were transmitted to us through these chromosomes, although a small amount of additional inheritance comes by way of some extranuclear cell organelles, such as the mitochondria, which code for many functions involved in their own replication. This additional inheritance is so small, however, that the NAS study effectively ignored it.

After meiosis, each germ cell will mature either into four sperm, in the male, or, in the female, into a single egg. The ensuing stages in the life of the sperm and the egg are discussed in previous chapters: what concerns us here is the array of processes which have resulted in a particular sperm or egg. Even the very sketchy account given above demonstrates the incredible complexity of our reproductive ecology. Any of these processes can go wrong or be damaged by the action of mutagens, with the resulting cells transmitting faulty instructions to the fertilized egg and, possibly, to the future generations which will branch out from it.

Such genetic effects can take place at the level of the gene itself, at the level of the chromosome, or at the level of the 'chromosome set' or 'genome', involving a change in the number of chromosomes. The question arises: are such mutations always harmful? 'It is commonly believed that mutations are almost invariably harmful,' the NAS report commented, 'whether they are genic, chromosomal or genomic. Some mutations have effects so minute as to be undetectable. Whether these are neutral or only nearly so is a matter of considerable discussion and experimentation. Nevertheless, we can say confidently that the overwhelming majority of mutations that have any overt effect at all are harmful.'

But what about beneficial mutations? 'A geneticist has to search to find examples of mutations that are clearly beneficial to the organism,' the NAS report concluded. 'Usually, these are found when the environment has been drastically altered. One example is DDT resistance in insects, but here it is worth noting that, in the absence of DDT, the resistance genes are usually mildly harmful. There are also a number of examples of benefit from the human viewpoint, but hardly from that of the animal in its wild state – for example, hornless cattle or non-brooding hens.'

Of course, some mutations must have proved useful – and must still prove useful – or we should never have evolved from the primordial slime. But, as the NAS report finally summed up, 'all organisms are the products of a long evolutionary history during which favorable genes have been preserved and deleterious genes eliminated by natural selection. A random change is more likely to make things worse than better.'

*

Let us consider some of the mutagenic effects we might expect to see at the three levels outlined above, to prepare the ground for a discussion of the ways in which we can pick out those mutations which have been induced by a chemical mutagen from those which are naturally occurring errors. We shall also be briefly considering the ways in which the health implications of such mutations are assessed, before turning to some of the gaps which remain in our understanding of the process of mutagenesis and of the environmental influences which promote it.

First, then, gene mutations. Genes, like chromosomes, occur in pairs. A gene which produces its characteristic effect when only one of its type is present is called a dominant gene, while a recessive gene is one which requires both genes to be of the same type. If a mutant gene is recessive, hundreds of generations may pass before it encounters another like itself and is expressed. If it were otherwise, the offspring of cousins would always be defective. A dominant gene, by contrast, will tend to be expressed in the generation immediately following that in which it first occurs.

Chromosomal mutations produce their effect largely by upsetting the balance of the genes transmitted, resulting in unusual combinations of genes, while genomic mutations lead to abnormal chromosome numbers. A surplus or shortage of any chromosome results in abnormalities, most of which have an adverse effect on the recipient's chances of survival. More than one third of all spontaneous abortions, it has been estimated, are caused either by chromosomal or by genomic mutations.

'The range of mutational effects is so wide,' the NAS study argued, 'and the future distribution of these effects so unpredictable in time and severity that it is impossible to make any convincing quantitative judgement of their total impact. However, the impact can be separated into two components, not entirely distinct, but sufficiently so to make the classification useful: dominant gene mutations and chromosomal mutations whose manifestation is confined to the first half-dozen generations after the mutation occurs; and mutations with very mild individual effects (such as those which cause a small increase in blood pressure) and recessive mutations whose effects are greatly diluted by time and whose effects on a single generation are much too small to measure.' The cut-off point most frequently adopted in mutagenicity research, and adopted for the purposes of the NAS study, involves focusing on those genetic effects which are thought likely to emerge in the first half-dozen generations.

A basic problem here is that none of us is genetically perfect. As the NAS study put it, 'the incidence of genetic impairment is 100 per cent. None of us is without some genetic deficiency and all of us will die, mostly from a cause that includes a genetic component.' It has been estimated, for example, that between 5 and 10 per cent of all human conceptions are chromosomally abnormal, and a high proportion of the chromosomal defects which result in genetic imbalance prove lethal long before the affected child is born. They are a major cause of spontaneous abortions or miscarriages. This fact, clearly, implies that until we are able to study the genetic make-up of a high proportion of such aborted foetuses, we shall continue to miss a very large component of the total mutational load in our populations.

Another problem is that even if we could distinguish between naturally occurring mutations and those which are being caused by environmental mutagens, it may be almost impossible to pinpoint the particular mutagen responsible. We are all exposed, throughout our lives, to chemicals and other agents which, in certain circumstances, can be carcinogenic, teratogenic or mutagenic. Some of these are highly dangerous and some border on the innocuous. Of course, this task may prove easier in the workplace, where, increasingly, records of exposure to particular chemicals are kept, but the general population is rarely aware of the potential threat. How many of us keep a record of the food additives we have consumed, for example, or of the hair dyes and other similar products we may have used?

If, knowingly or not, we have been exposed to a mutagen, we may still be hard-pressed to pinpoint its effect. We may be run down by a bus long before the mutation has had time to take effect or, more importantly for the research scientist, we may miss the effect in the crowd of symptoms and ailments we all suffer as we grow older. Exposure to a mutagen is highly unlikely to result in a predictable health effect in the same way that a virus or heavy metal might. Looking further afield, any long-distance, inheritable mutations are currently likely to escape notice. How many of us know what work our grandparents or great-grandparents did, let alone what chemicals they were exposed to in the course of their uncharted lives?

As far as health effects are concerned, exposure to a mutagen would typically produce a 'pulse' of mutations in the generations immediately following that (or those) exposed. Typically, too, those mutations which generate the most serious health effects would tend to produce their damage sooner rather than later – and would tend to be eliminated in a few generations. Milder mutations, by contrast, would not affect their recipients' survival as badly, and therefore might be expected to produce health effects over a much longer period of time.

Anyone reading through the literature on mutations must be struck by how much we still have to learn. As the NAS study put it, 'the health consequences of deleterious mutation in populations are poorly understood, despite the large effort that has been expended in the study of mutation. Spontaneous mutation rates are known only roughly, the forces that maintain or alter gene frequencies in populations are not well understood, and the relative impacts of different types of mutations are obscure.'

It is known, however, that chromosomal and genomic mutations tend to produce severe dominant effects, with the result that a very high proportion of those fertilized eggs affected actually die during the early stages of embryonic development. If the embryo survives, it tends to be seriously compromised. The impact of point mutations (mutations which affect only one or a few DNA base points in a gene), by contrast, tends to depend on which gene product is affected and to what extent. In some cases, no gene product (such as an amino acid) may actually be produced, with the impact depending on how important that missing product is in the normal human body. Alternatively, a defective or different gene product may be produced, with the impact here depending on how important the defective or replaced gene product is – and how much damage the mutation-induced product can cause in its own right.

Chromosome abnormalities are almost certainly the most clear-cut of human mutations, accounting for at least sixty different conditions in those children surviving beyond birth. The best known health effects of such abnormalities include the Down's, Edwards, Patau and Klinefelter syndromes. Studies of the chromosomes of 56,000 newborn infants in many countries showed a frequency of abnormalities of about one in 150 and, on the basis of studies of foetuses lost through spontaneous abortion, it seems likely that at least 6 per cent of all early human conceptions leading to a recognizable pregnancy are chromosomally abnormal in some way. It is also estimated that about 90 per cent of chromosomally abnormal foetuses are rejected as spontaneous abortions.

As far as defects and diseases due to defective genes are concerned, the picture is even more complicated. Such genetically induced conditions in the newborn range from cystic fibrosis and mental retardation through childhood blindness and deafness to Tay-Sachs disease – which is an example of the ethnic variation in the incidence of such conditions. Among Ashkenazi Jews, Tay-Sachs disease appears with a frequency of between 17 and 40 births per 100,000, compared with a frequency of about 0.1 per 100,000 in the non-Ashkenazi population. Other conditions in which genetic factors are known to play an important role include cyclothymia (which shows up in about 4 births per 1,000), epilepsy (5 births per 1,000), diabetes mellitus (3–10 births per 1,000) and schizophrenia (8–10 births per 1,000).

If one considers the overall contribution of genetic factors to the incidence of human disease, it looks as though they are responsible for disorders in perhaps 4 to 5 per cent of live births. Clearly, with such an extraordinarily 'noisy' background of mutations and defects, it is often extremely difficult, where it is possible at all, to distinguish 'blips' in the statistics which might be attributable to chemical or other mutagens.

And what happens when we start to move out from some of the known, fairly potent mutagens to look at some of the less powerful? It is entirely possible that severe mutations are the tip of a mutational iceberg. If we consider those mutations which have a relatively mild effect, which occur at relatively high rates and which are inefficiently selected out of human populations by natural selection, tests in *Drosophila* (fruit-flies) and other species suggest that such milder mutations may outnumber severe-effect mutations by at least 10 to 1. 'The human situation is not understood,' the NAS study confirmed, 'but it is possible that, for every severe mutation detected by laboratory test systems, 20 or more mildly deleterious mutations also occur.' Such mutations clearly affect the health of both wild and experimental fruit-flies, but the question remains: do they affect ours? The answer, ultimately, will almost certainly be that they do.

Many mutagens will probably be discovered almost accidentally, but the chances of discovering them will clearly fall off as we begin to look for those which cause milder mutations in test systems. Genetic toxicology may make some totally unexpected advances in our lifetimes, but the task ahead is clearly a daunting one.

Another problem is that while we might invest enormous resources in a screening programme designed to identify potential mutagens among the phenomenal number of pure chemicals now in use, mutagens often come as just one component in complex mixtures such as industrial effluents. The testing of such mixtures is obviously going to be of considerable importance in pinpointing and controlling mutation risks, but teasing out and evaluating the culprit chemicals and any interactions which may be taking place between them is not going to be easy.

This is not to say, of course, that it is impossible to test environmental samples for mutagenicity: indeed, a great deal of work is already being done in just this field. George Hoffman, who was involved in the NAS study, pointed out, 'Mutagenicity studies of environmental samples require a broad range of techniques for the collection of samples, their extraction or concentration, and their fractionation to characterize their mutagenic components.' While they can be (and are being) improved, much of the necessary technology already exists.

Among the complex mixtures that have been tested to date are: drinking water and swimming pool water; industrial emissions and effluent; municipal sewage sludge; welding fumes; vehicle emissions; the emissions from plants burning wood, peat and oil; fossil fuels, including shale oils; photocopy toners; typewriter ribbon extracts; coal fly ash; coffee and tea; cooked meat and fish; smoke from charred meat; and tobacco smoke. So, if you smoke, have barbecues, type for a living or simply breathe the city air, someone somewhere probably has information on the extent to which what your are doing may be endangering your genes – although that information needs to be looked at with a highly critical eye. With such a variety of test systems and procedures, it is hardly surprising that a particular chemical can show up as a mutagen one day and obtain a clean bill of health from another laboratory or another test the next.

Logically, too, if mutagens can sometimes reinforce each other, producing unexpected, non-additive (or synergistic) health effects, so we might expect them to cancel each other out on occasion. In other cases, the activity of a mutagen may be depressed by a non-mutagenic substance. An example of this emerged when one research team added a polyaromatic fraction from tar sand to a bacterial test system which already contained the known mutagen

2-aminoanthracene – and discovered that its mutagenicity disappeared, at least as far as that particular test system was concerned.

The existence of such 'anti-mutagens' has raised the idea in some people's minds of producing a pill against mutagens, although the NAS team dismissed the possibility. 'Perhaps it will be possible to counter the effects of an increase in environmental mutagens by lowering the spontaneous mutation rate, which must be due in part to chemical influences,' the team suggested, imagining the use of yet more chemicals to control the mutagenic effects of those we already use. But, it concluded, 'It is not likely that a pill that reduces the mutation rate and possibly reduces carcinogenesis as a byproduct (and has no adverse side-effects) will suddenly appear.'

Indeed. But the NAS team did identify two ways in which the reduction of the mutation rate could be approached. 'The first,' it said, 'is to identify substances that counteract known mutagens. Such chemicals have been found, but they might have an opposite effect elsewhere – e.g. converting non-mutagens into mutagens. Intermediate metabolism (and especially toxification and detoxification) is so complicated that it is difficult to be sure that one understands all the effects of an added chemical. The second approach involves direct chemical intervention in the mutation process itself. A number of processes are known to affect mutation and pre-mutational damage, but it is also possible that the bulk of mutation is caused by errors in DNA repair. It may be possible to interfere with error-prone systems while keeping repair error-free. However, such treatment may well increase cell death, which itself may cause harm that offsets a reduction in mutation.'

A lot of ifs and buts. As usual, it looks as though it will make a great deal more sense to try to prevent mutations rather than try to control them chemically once they have begun to surface. There are those who see the lack of direct, incontrovertible evidence of mutations induced in humans by environmental mutagens as reason enough for dropping the subject entirely. So far, however, genetic toxicology has been fairly well supported, particularly in the United States. As Donald Clive of Burroughs Wellcome's genetic toxicology laboratory has put it, 'like exobiology [the study of extra-terrestrial life-forms], environmental germ-cell mutagenesis is a subject of study without a subject to study. Unlike exobiology, however, environmental mutagenesis is well funded.'

One possible reason why we do not appear to be swamped with chemically induced mutations may be that the womb (or, as the scientist would put it, the uterine environment) is a far more sophisticated system for weeding out such problems at an early stage than we had ever suspected. We have seen that many foetuses which are aborted have been found to have chromosomal or other genetic damage. But we have also seen that the womb is far from perfect in dealing with the effects of such teratogens as mercury and thalidomide: why should we expect it to be any better at picking off mutations in the unborn?

Simultaneously, modern medicine is making tremendous advances which are enabling doctors to save foetuses which would otherwise have been aborted and premature babies which would otherwise have died shortly after birth. With the evidence before us, we must at least admit the possibility that a significant proportion of these medical rescues will turn out to have ensured the survival of children whose genetic make-up, for whatever reason, is flawed in some way.

The strong links between mutagenesis and carcinogenesis have both spurred the development of new generations of test systems and ensured that this work attracts funding. We may not all be particularly concerned about what happens six generations down the line from us, but which of us can say that the threat of cancer leaves us unmoved? The links between carcinogenesis and mutagenesis are explored in Chapter 7, but first we turn to the legislative dikes which have been erected in recent years between our burgeoning chemical technology and our all-too-vulnerable reproductive systems. And it is worth casting our minds back to 1980, when Ronald Reagan captured the White House, to provide the political backdrop to some of the shifts in the public's perception of environmental problems which have arisen in the intervening years. After a period in the political doldrums, environmental concerns have leaped back up the agenda – with the control of carcinogens, mutagens and teratogens very near the top of the list.

CHAPTER SIX

THE
VANISHING
THRESHOLD

'They took a lesson from the Vietnam war: declare victory and pull out.' This was the reaction of one legal expert when he heard that the Reagan administration was going to disband its controversial Task Force on Regulatory Relief. The news, which was broken at a hastily arranged press conference while Congress was out of session, was seen by many as evidence that President Reagan's campaign to dismantle or draw the teeth of much of the environmental and other legislation passed in the 1970s was running out of steam. The United States was already gearing up for the 1984 election and, said one White House aide, 'the political dividends aren't very high'. In 1980, things had looked different.

The Task Force, which had been headed by Vice President George Bush, had been the nerve centre of the campaign to 'get the regulators off the backs of the people', to use a phrase which surfaced as Ronald Reagan's challenge to President Carter moved into top gear. Industry, both in America and elsewhere, had long complained about the financial and administrative burdens imposed by environmental, health and safety legislation, but the Republican victory in 1980 heralded a major series of attacks on such bodies as the Environmental Protection Agency (EPA).

'Environmentalists tremble' read one headline in *Science* shortly after the election of Mr Reagan as President. If they did, they had good reason to do so: the ex-actor had been, to put it mildly, an uninspiring candidate as far as environmental issues went. At one stage he asserted that trees were a major source of air pollution. And he also claimed that air pollution was at last under control – on the same day that a pea-soup photochemical smog prevented his plane from landing at Los Angeles airport.

One of President Reagan's first acts on taking office was to impose a sixty-day freeze on new regulations, although on the environmental front only twenty relatively minor regulations were affected, and the three most important of these were already the subject of court orders forcing the EPA to implement them during the sixty-day period. None the less, the moratorium was a sign of things to come. The new administration also immediately reversed President Carter's ban on the export of hazardous products whose sale was restricted in the United States.

The Republicans took their lead from a crop of reports arguing that regulation was almost an un-American activity. One conservative think-tank, the Heritage Foundation, had published a report which was sharply critical of the EPA. Arguing that 'the EPA has not been reluctant to support fears raised by persons on mere allegations', the Foundation concluded that 'the public are ill-served by "science by innuendo"'. The report, which also accused the EPA of designing its research programmes to support 'pre-conceived regulatory policy', was seen by many environmentalists as a blueprint for the gutting of the EPA. Their fears proved well-founded.

The outgoing administrator of the EPA, Douglas Costle, had this to say about the likely future trend in environmental policy under the Republican regime: 'There are fundamental demographic changes that we're going through in this country. As you look at the polls,' he continued, 'the young people feel a lot more strongly about environmental issues than the age group that will be represented in the government leaders in the next four years. I don't think society is going to permit a turning back of the clock.' Significantly, a public opinion poll carried out at the time of the Afghanistan crisis (not a time when the environment was uppermost in most people's minds) showed that, while public concern about environmental issues had lessened somewhat from a peak on Earth Day in 1970, there was continuing strong support for environmental protection. To take just one question in the survey, respondents were asked to consider the following statement: 'Protecting the environment is so important that requirements and standards cannot be too high, and continuing improvement must be made *regardless* of cost.' Over 40 per cent of the sample chose this statement rather than milder or anti-environmental alternatives.

Costle was not alone in believing that the appointment of a hardline Republican, David Stockman, as director of the Office of Management and Budget (OMB) was an ill omen. 'OMB can kill this agency,' he warned, 'and you won't see any scars – except that you won't see much coming out either.' At that time, the various trade associations in Washington, DC, were spending over $4 billion a year, half of which was going on staff costs, to ensure that they got their views across to Congress and the public. But the departing Costle saw ground for some optimism in the attitudes of a solid core of forward-thinking industrialists.

'Most corporate chief executive officers,' he suggested, 'tend to be moderate-conservative pragmatists, underlining the word *pragmatists*. They want certainty and they want rationality in the process, but they're not thinking: "Let's just turn back the clock." There are some that are, obviously, but they also tend to be very smart and realize that if they push back the pendulum too far, too fast, it will spring back at them that much faster.' Indeed, I recall talking to one American chief executive in Washington at the time. His concern was that the pendulum had already been pushed back so far that next time it would 'smash through the wall of the clock'.

Writing from Washington in the summer of 1981, I reported: 'Walking around the corridors of 722 Jackson Place, the home of the Council on Environmental Quality, is rather like walking around a ghost town.' On 19 March that year, the CEQ's then acting chairman, Mr Malcolm Baldwin, was instructed to fire fifty-eight of the CEQ's fifty-nine employees – himself included. Mr Baldwin, a lifelong Republican, was very much taken by surprise, particularly since he had supported Governor Reagan's campaign for the Presidency.

'The CEQ's incoming chairman,' I noted, 'is Mr Al Hill. Although he has been a purveyor of bathroom fixtures for the last seven years, since his failure to win a seat in the California State Assembly elections of 1974, Mr Hill does have a certain understanding of environmental issues. Early in the 1970s, he worked in the Californian Resources Agency and then served as deputy director of the State's Department of Conservation. It could have been worse.'

Over at the EPA, it *was* worse. Indeed, a leader in the *New York*

Times reacted to the ensuing chaos in the Agency with the following words: 'Seldom since the Emperor Caligula appointed his horse a consul has there been so wide a gulf between authority and competence. Mr Reagan's EPA appointees brought almost no relevant experience to their jobs. His administrator, Anne Burford, was a telephone company attorney and two-term legislator who learned about environmental issues fighting Clean Air Act provisions in Colorado.'

Back in Colorado, some of these appointees had actually been known in the Colorado Legislature as the 'House Crazies'. Members of a band of militant conservatives who came to power in 1979, they had fought against controls on air pollution and toxic waste dumps, against programmes designed to immunize schoolchildren against mumps and measles, and against such schemes as one designed to teach the handicapped to ski. 'People called us "crazies" because when we started out everybody said we were crazy to think we could change the government,' said one former activist. 'They were wrong.'

Indeed they were. Anne Gorsuch, who became Anne Burford when she married another staunch Republican, Robert Burford, at the height of the campaign to remove her from office, had a strong ally in James Watt, President Reagan's choice as Secretary of the Interior. 'How many times do I have to read about the fox guarding the chicken house,' Watt complained shortly after his appointment, 'or of Dracula in charge of the blood bank?' Cast as the villain of the piece, Watt faced an unprecedented reaction from environmentalists – with even the relatively staid Sierra Club coordinating a nationwide campaign calling on the President to fire the erstwhile Denver lawyer.

While Watt may have felt himself misjudged, he certainly was a choice guaranteed to rile environmentalists. Not only had he been an ardent anti-environmentalist in his days with the Chamber of Commerce's Natural Resources Committee and Environmental Pollution Panel (where he played an active part in the Chamber's lobbying against clean air and clear water legislation), and with the Mountain States Legal Foundation (which defended the rights of its member companies who, as Friends of the Earth put it, were 'like a *Who's Who* of western resource developers'), but he had also been a leading light in the so-called 'sagebrush rebellion'. This involved a coalition of ranchers, miners, power companies and other natural resource interests which wanted to return millions of acres of federal land, much of it under the control of the Department of the Interior, to state and private ownership.

Given that the federal government owned something like 30 per cent of the State of Montana at the time, and an extraordinary 87 per cent of Nevada, it is not difficult to see why there was resentment. Some 12,400 miles of America's coastline and 770 million acres were in government ownership. But the new Secretary of the Interior's comments seemed calculated to raise environmental hackles as he moved to allow oil drilling and other development on such land. 'We don't know how many generations we can count on before Jesus returns,' said Watt, a religious fundamentalist. 'My responsibility is to follow the Scriptures, which call upon us to occupy the land until He does.'

A symptom of these political shifts was the administration's reaction to the growing acid rain problem. Just as it was launching 'Project Democracy', designed to promote in other countries such American values as freedom of speech, the Justice Department was labelling as 'political propaganda' three films made in Canada. Two of these dealt with the environmental risks of acid rain, while the third was a documentary on nuclear war. The Justice Department was insisting that they should only be shown with a statement of official disapproval – and that the Department should receive a list of all those who rented the films.

'It sounds like something you would expect from the Soviet Union, not the United States,' retorted the Canadian Environment Minister, John Roberts. Canada blames the United States for the acidification of many of its lakes, charging that the sulphur dioxide released from industrial smokestacks returns to the ground some distance away as sulphuric acid – a charge which was also being levelled against countries such as Britain by Norway and Sweden.

But perhaps the most blatant perversion of an environmental programme centred on the $1.6 billion 'Superfund', set up in the wake of such scandals as the Love Canal disaster. Drawing on contributions from waste-producers, with costs recouped from violators, the Superfund gave the EPA the money and authority to deal with the toxic waste dumps which environmentalists dubbed 'ticking time bombs'. Yet, as the ticking became louder, it was only too clear that the Reagan administration was doing everything in its power to delay the clean-up process.

It took several years for the EPA to identify the 418 sites thought to be most dangerous: by early 1983 it had dealt with precisely five of these. Two Congressional sub-committees, attracted to the EPA by the controversy surrounding Anne Burford, closed in like sharks on the scent of blood. They charged that the EPA's new management was making 'sweetheart deals' with industry which let polluters off the hook. When Burford refused to turn over subpoenaed documents relating to 160 of the sites, she was cited for contempt of Congress. The ensuing allegations of perjury, conflict of interest and manipulation of funds triggered three more House of Representatives sub-committees and a Senate committee to join in the hunt.

Despite efforts by the President to shore up Burford and others, using executive privilege to impede the investigations, the evidence already in the public domain was too damning. The press was full of allegations that through the night secret papers had been fed into shredders in the beleaguered Agency; that witnesses were lying under oath; that 'whistle-blowers' had been harassed and erasures made in some of the subpoenaed documents. The first victim was Rita Lavelle, who had overseen the hazardous waste programmes, and a chain of resignations and sackings eventually led to the sacking of Burford herself.

But the damage had been done. The EPA's resources had been halved at a time when its responsibilities were doubling. Its enforcement efforts were wrecked by constant internal reorganizations, and its morale was at an all-time low. Even some industry people were finding it all too much. 'There's a bizarre quality to the whole place,' said one lobbyist working for a major chemical company. 'It's turned into a never-never-land of rumor, innuendo and constant bureaucratic upheaval.' Things had got so bad, said William Hedeman, who was head of the toxic waste clean-up programme, that 'loyal, hardworking employees are even ashamed to admit to their friends or neighbours they work at the agency'.

The American experience, as usual, simply took a trend to extremes. No one disputes that the United States had introduced an unprecedented succession of powerful and sweeping new regulations since the late 1960s, among them the Clean Air and Clean Water Acts, the National Environmental Policy Act, the Noise Control Act, the Marine Protection, Research and Sanctuaries Act, the Federal Insecticide and Rodenticide Act, the Toxic Substances Control Act, and the Resource Conservation and Recovery Act.

And there was a growing body of opinion that the time had come for the whole process of environmental regulation and enforcement to be streamlined or 'fine-tuned'. Indeed, the incoming administration used such words to describe its intentions. But, like the knights who assassinated Thomas à Becket in 1170, the Crazies took their instructions a good deal too literally. President Reagan, like Henry II, found himself having to do penance for the resulting damage.

The 1970s had certainly been a busy period for environmental legislators. When the Organization for Economic Co-operation and Development (OECD) published its first State of the Environment report in 1979, it included a listing of the new legislation passed in OECD countries during the decade. The take-off point in many countries came in the years following the United Nations' Stockholm Conference on the Human Environment, held in 1972. The period from 1972 to 1976 represents something of a 'hump' in any graph plotting this outpouring of new laws and controls.

This growth in environmental legislation was paralleled (and then spurred on) by a secondary growth cycle in the body politic. Soon every OECD country had at least an embryonic institutional framework for dealing with environmental problems. Japan had its Environment Agency, the United States its EPA, Switzerland its Federal Environmental Protection Bureau, West Germany its Federal Environment Agency and the UK its Department of the Environment, to name but a few. Taiwan's Bureau of Environmental Protection, founded in 1982, was clearly something of a late starter.

Environmental protection, as I discovered when I carried out a study for the OECD's own Environment Directorate in 1977, had been among the fastest-growing sectors of public expenditure in the industrialized western economies. Japan, a late starter in the industrialization stakes, made up for lost time – in the wake of such disasters as the mercury pollution of Minamata Bay – and displayed a spectacular growth in the proportion of its gross national product devoted to environmental clean-up and protection. The Japanese experience was extraordinary in a number of ways, but it is interesting to note that a report by the Battelle Institute, carried out for the West German Federal Ministry of the Interior in 1975, concluded that some 50 per cent of the pollution control expenditure ever made in West Germany had been made in the five years from 1970 to 1975.

The evolution of environmental law was so rapid that even environmental legislators had difficulty in keeping track of developments. Inevitably, too, some of this legislation proved unworkable or misconceived. Part of the problem was that much of it was drafted at breakneck speed, generally in a headlong attempt to close the stable door after a succession of bolted horses.

There is much in American environmental law, for example, that smacks of emergency measures, of older federal, state and local pollution laws extended precipitately into applications for which they were never designed. And one set of controls has often triggered the next generation of problems. The Clean Air Act aggravated Canada's acid rain problems as industrialists built ever-taller chimneys, dispersing their emissions over ever-greater areas. At the same time, the Act forced industry to impound its toxic wastes in pits, ponds and lagoons, from which they all too often percolated down to contaminate underground water resources (often called 'groundwater').

These problems, in turn, led to second-generation legislation such as the Resource Conservation and Recovery Act. But all the time the costs were mounting. Total environmental expenditures, the US Commerce Department told President Reagan, amounted to about $48.5 billion in 1979, representing in constant dollars a 29 per cent increase over the position in 1972. And, according to the CEQ, the cumulative costs in the period from 1977 to 1988 would amount to $735 *billion*, using 1979 dollars and assuming no new laws.

It is easy to see why the Republicans were keen to cut back on environmental regulations. Once again, there was a great deal of talk about 'cost-benefit analysis' or, in simpler terms, about getting environmental value for money spent. However, as Costle put it at the time, 'for every hundred people running around this town screaming "cost-benefit", there probably aren't three of them who've ever done it. The problem,' he stressed, 'isn't with the concept – the concept sounds great; it has a lovely rhetorical ring. But just wait until you sit down and actually try to do one when you can't even adequately quantify the costs. We found in looking at the six most expensive rule-makings at EPA that both industry and the government overestimated the costs of compliance by very substantial orders of magnitude in four cases out of six.'

The American approach to pollution control, based as it was as much on the opinions of lawyers as on the research results produced by scientists, was bound to provoke a reaction from those who had to foot the bill for the laundering of the national environment. And this reaction, in turn, forced environmental scientists and regulators to consider different control options. The chairman of the National Academy of Sciences' environmental studies board, Dr John Cantlon, encapsulated the lessons of the late 1970s in the following words: 'I do not think that all the census work that I have seen indicates that people are willing to give up clean air or clean water. But they are more willing than before to ask the question whether the cost-effectiveness of certain regulations are defensible.'

Two new approaches formulated around that time were the 'bubble concept' and the 'emission offset policy', both designed to cut the cost to industry of environmental clean-up operations. The emission offset policy meant that new industry could move into areas with very restrictive pollution controls, provided that existing industrial polluters could be persuaded (usually with cash) to make a compensating reduction in the pollution *they* generated. The second cost-cutting innovation, the bubble concept, may have sounded like common sense to British industrialists and environmentalists, but represented a radical departure from normal EPA practice. The standard EPA approach to controlling emissions or effluents from a factory or other industrial plant had involved specifying a pollution emission standard for *each* smokestack, vent or other pollution source on a given site. The new approach, by contrast, involved dealing with pollution in relation to the plant's emissions as a whole – by enclosing it in an imaginary bubble, which was then considered to be the pollution source to be controlled.

Under the previous set-up, a large steel mill, oil refinery or chemical plant would have had to meet forty or fifty different pollution standards, representing a major financial burden on the affected company. The new policy meant that a refinery which was paying perhaps $50 a ton to control smog-promoting hydrocarbons evaporating from storage tanks, compared to an outlay of thousands of dollars per ton spent on the control of pollution coming from leaks, defective equipment or other 'fugitive emissions', was permitted to save money by concentrating on meeting the overall standard by the cheapest route.

The basic idea was to find ways in which industry could be encouraged to be an eager partner in efforts to control pollution, generally by appealing to the profit motive. In particular, the EPA wanted to stimulate innovation in pollution control technology, believing that the existing methods were often primitive and expensive.

In the event, the reaction turned out to be an over-reaction. The EPA's Republican appointees tried to go too far too fast, trampling on too many toes in the process. Some of them also went off in completely the wrong direction. They encouraged companies to carry out superficial, essentially cosmetic, clean-ups at problem toxic waste dumps rather than requiring a thoroughly professional operation. Some suffered from acute conflicts of interest. Rita Lavelle, who ultimately ended up in court, where she was found guilty of perjury, took part in decisions involving a California toxic waste dump – even though her previous employer, Aerojet Liquid Rocket Co., was under investigation because of the part it had played in making the dump one of the most dangerous in the country. It was also alleged that Superfund clean-up resources had been held back from states which, like Governor Jerry Brown's California, were politically out of line with the Reagan administration.

The sacking of Anne Burford and the later resignation of James Watt reflected the considerable political clout which the environment lobby could still deploy. It also left President Reagan with the thorny problem of choosing a successor. He eventually picked William Ruckelshaus, the EPA's first administrator. Ruckelshaus, who was a staunch Republican and who resigned a $220,000-a-year job with the timber products company Weyerhaeuser to take up the $70,000 EPA post, was an inspired choice. Known as 'Mr Clean', he had built a reputation as something of a white knight, having taken a stand against President Nixon at the time of the Watergate scandal even though he owed his original EPA appointment to Nixon. Taking over the EPA for the second time, he announced that there would be 'no hit lists, no political decisions and no sweetheart deals'. The reference to 'hit lists' was effectively a promise to drop another practice which had been rampant under Mrs Burford: any scientist who sat on an EPA advisory panel and offended right-wing sensibilities was listed as 'a menace' or 'pure ecology type' – and dumped.

Working in the new EPA, said Ruckelshaus, would be like

working 'in a fish bowl'. EPA officials should think of everything they said or did, even behind closed doors, 'as if it were on a billboard'. But, while many environmentalists were enormously relieved to have him in Mrs Burford's stead, there were those who noted that while at Weyerhaeuser he had repeatedly written to members of Congress urging them to relax the Clean Air Act. A decision made in 1979, while he was still at the EPA, to permit power stations in Georgia to shoot air pollution up into the atmosphere through tall smokestacks had earned him the title 'God-father of Acid Rain'. Weyerhaeuser, too, had been urging the EPA to allow Dow Chemical to resume sales of 2,4,5-T, the controversial herbicide.

Despite all these problems, there were still those who felt that the United States was streets ahead in environmental protection – simply because it had the EPA. As chairman of the UK branch of Friends of the Earth, Des Wilson accepted that the EPA was 'less than ideal' and 'in its present form is clearly not a model for other countries to follow. But,' he concluded, 'the *idea* is.' The Agency's strength, in Wilson's view, had been its complete independence, at least in theory, and its authority to produce and enforce regulations to control pollution. Its weakness had been that its top officials were political appointees and as such tended to reflect current administration policy – and were 'vulnerable to its whims'.

The EPA's greatest advantage had been that it operated in the United States, which had a Freedom of Information Act. When dealing with particular pollution problems, the EPA tended to use open hearings and published all the evidence it received. This approach provided a striking contrast to that adopted even in such relatively forward-thinking countries as Britain.

'There is an inherent flaw in the British governmental structure,' Wilson suggested when lobbying for a UK equivalent of the EPA and of the Freedom of Information Act, 'and that flaw is the reason for our poor environmental record. Whitehall and Westminster crumble in the face of the industrial lobby. The system isn't working because environmental and public health protection do not warrant sufficient priority – and there is a massive bias within the British bureaucracy towards the status quo and towards short-term economic factors. There is also an arrogance that allows it to believe it knows best and that it can trample over evidence that is contrary to its view.'

Environmentalists such as Wilson could point to the astonishing delays achieved by the industrial lobbies in the implementation of such central pieces of legislation as the 1974 Control of Pollution Act. Indeed, at times it seemed that the only factor which was ensuring that the UK Department of the Environment inched forward occasionally was the country's membership of the EEC. The impact of the EEC's environmental directives has varied from one member state to the next and, like that of national legislation, from one industry to the next, but few industrialists would dispute that the Commission of the European Communities has become one of the major regulatory powerhouses.

One feature of the Commission's approach which has dismayed some industrialists and delighted many environmentalists has been its unusual receptiveness to the environmental case. The Commission has also tended to go for the American approach in environmental protection. Britain, in consequence, has tended to stick out like a sore thumb in successive debates about pressing environmental issues. The Department of the Environment has enthused about its 'pragmatic' stance on such issues and has emphasized the central role of the 'gentleman's agreement' in achieving improved environmental standards in, say, the pesticides, detergent or packaging industries. But this approach has its weaknesses, and it has failed to recruit the sympathies of most European environmentalists. As one Italian put it, it is not so much that 'there are no gentlemen in the rest of Europe'. Rather, voluntary self-regulation is quite simply not part of the political or cultural tradition in many European countries.

So the Commission continued to draft new legislation which, like the Sixth Amendment to the EEC's 1967 Directive on the classification, packaging and labelling of dangerous substances, has forced industry throughout the region to carry out growing batteries of health and ecological tests on the chemicals they wish to bring to market.

Under the terms of the Directive, a manufacturer or importer of a new chemical of which more than one tonne is likely to be sold in a normal year has to notify the relevant control agencies (in the case of the UK, the Department of the Environment and the Health and Safety Executive) before it goes on sale. This notification must alert the control agencies to the chemical's basic properties, impurities, toxic effects, intended uses and any recommended precautions to be adopted in its handling, packaging and ultimate disposal. A government can demand additional information and safety tests if more than 10 tonnes are likely to be sold, and these tests become mandatory when sales of more than 100 tonnes a year are being considered. Above 1,000 tonnes a year, the manufacturer or importer will be required to supply even more information, including evidence that the product does not cause cancer or birth defects.

A major problem is that while some control authorities have argued that the national legislation implementing the EEC Directive contains many loopholes, cuts in the staffing and resources available to such agencies have raised doubts whether they can even handle the information they now receive. One top scientist at the Department of the Environment, Dr Norman King, was unusually outspoken for a British civil servant. If the EEC notification scheme was to work, he suggested, 'a more active role must be assumed by the notification team'. To ensure that the information received could be used as part of an early warning system, he said, he needed more than the handful of staff he had been given. But in the prevailing economic climate he would probably have counted himself lucky even to keep those people he already had.

Yet Britain, despite its constant arguments with the Commission, has been among the most conscientious countries as far as actually implementing EEC legislation is concerned. Others, such as Italy, have implemented little. Some attempts have been made to assess the overall effectiveness of the EEC's environmental legislation, including a study carried out by the European Environmental Policy Programme (EEPP), a joint venture between the Institute for European Environmental Policy and the International Institute for Environment and Development. But the EEPP found it very difficult indeed to pull together a coherent picture, often because the Commission had not yet published the necessary information. And the Commission, in turn, complained that member states had been far too slow in compiling their own state-of-the-environment reports, on which the EEC's assessments would be based. Indeed, while William Ruckelshaus was settling into his seat at the EPA, the Commission was threatening to take seven EEC countries to court because of their failure to complete reports on toxic waste disposal. Only Britain, Luxembourg and West Germany had obliged at that stage, and the Commission was complaining that of the three submitted, 'some are inadequate'.

But some problem chemicals have certainly been effectively controlled through international cooperation, including polychlorinated biphenyls (PCBs). A decision taken in 1973 by the Council of the Organization for Economic Co-operation and Development (OECD) was, in retrospect, a watershed in the international control of the environmental hazards linked with the use and disposal of industrial chemicals. The decision, which launched concerted international action to deal with the threat posed by the widespread dissemination of PCBs in the environment, was in turn an important catalyst for the enactment of the new generation of chemical regulations.

The ecological problems caused by PCBs stemmed from some of the very properties which made them commercially attractive: in particular, their chemical stability and their solubility in other organic liquids. This stability meant that the PCB molecule persisted in the environment for an unusually long time, while its solubility led to its entering the food chain. By a process of bioaccumulation, it found its way into the tissues of a wide variety of wildlife, and into human tissues.

Accidental exposures of people in Japan and America to high doses of PCBs resulted in outbreaks of skin disease, blindness and gastro-intestinal illness, while improved analytical methods began to pick up traces in cow's milk, in plastic-wrapped chicken and in food wrapping made from recycled copying paper. In a number of cases, exposure to PCBs was found to result in reproductive failure in wildlife species.

As the evidence continued to accumulate, discussions took place between governments and industry. By 1972, the year before the OECD decision, five of the six PCB manufacturers in the various countries had voluntarily reduced production to the levels needed to support demand in a small number of approved uses, typically in closed systems such as power transformers and heat-transfer systems. Since 1973, the production of PCBs has fallen sharply. By 1980, it had been reduced by more than 60 per cent (from 44,276 tonnes to 16,586). Imports also fell dramatically, and soon the use of PCBs was more or less restricted to just two applications: transformers and capacitors.

Environmental monitoring has not shown an equally dramatic fall in levels of PCB in the environment, probably because of the molecule's intrinsic stability. And the fact that large quantities are still being stored in some countries, pending the construction of suitable incinerators, suggests that there is little room for complacency. At the same time, the economic climate has meant that 'cowboy' toxic waste contractors, who offer to get rid of such waste on the cheap, have been quietly coming back into business.

'In the last year we've lost 15 per cent of our chemical treatment business,' said Dr Arthur Coleman of Re-Chem International, a UK company which runs a number of incineration plants around the country. 'Some of this is due to the recession, but a lot more is due to industry switching back to landfill and cutting corners.' Coleman was convinced that 'Saturday morning specials' were back on the road, dumping loads of toxic waste on council refuse tips when the inspectors were at rest. 'We lost one contract for incinerating cutting fluid recently,' he said. 'The company said the fluid was going to a plant in Cambridgeshire for recycling. I know what's in the fluid and I don't believe there is anything worth recycling. And as far as we can discover there isn't a recovery plant anywhere in Cambridgeshire anyway.' Coleman should know about recycling: Re-Chem was originally set up to reclaim and recycle chemical wastes, as its name suggests, but the economics of recycling proved prohibitive.

Re-Chem, in fact, had earlier become embroiled in the Kepone story. Opening a debate in the House of Commons on the company's plan to incinerate the Kepone residues at its Pontypool plant, the MP for Pontypool, Leo Abse, stated that 'no one, certainly not one of my constituents, doubts the compelling necessity to have controlled waste disposal centres to deal with the problems of toxic waste disgorged by modern industry'. Re-Chem's plan to burn toxic wastes, however, had persuaded Mr Abse that its operations posed a threat to the community. He questioned whether the UK, which was only just getting around to clearing away some of the ravages imposed in Wales by the Industrial Revolution, should now become a 'receptacle for the excreta of American capitalism'.

In the event, the Kepone residues went down a salt mine in West Germany. Meanwhile, American companies have continued to export chemical wastes, with Mexico, Canada, Japan and a number of European countries taking in this toxic 'laundry'. Like the growing international trade in nuclear waste between those with nuclear power plants and those with reprocessing facilities, these transfrontier shipments of chemical waste may make economic sense but are not always popular in the receiving country.

Some countries have been left holding the toxic 'baby'. In 1980, a Mexican company run by an American, Clarence Nugent, dumped 5,000 tonnes of mercury-bearing wastes down an abandoned mine in Mexico. Nugent ended up serving two years in a Mexican gaol. He was simply unlucky. Elsewhere, the liquidation of such waste disposal companies as Riafield Ltd, which used to ship toxic wastes from the Netherlands to Britain, left other companies, including BP, with the embarrassing problem of having to dispose of waste shipments they had taken in from Riafield on a temporary basis.

The Netherlands was just recovering from the scandals of 1980 surrounding the Lekkerkerk waste disposal site when an even more serious problem emerged at Gouderak. The inhabitants of a ninety-six house estate were warned that it had been built on top of 135 tonnes of polycyclic aromatics, 0.11 tonnes of benzene, 14.6 tonnes of aldrin, dieldrin and endrin residues, and 13.2 tonnes of PCBs. Gouderak was built on reclaimed land which had been filled with household and industrial wastes. The disposal permits specifically excluded chemicals and oils, but Shell Nederland Chemie in Pernis admitted that despite this it had dumped residues from the production of the 'drin' pesticides.

It is tempting to attribute such problems to attitudes which have long since been consigned to the dustbin of history, but this would be unduly optimistic. At the time that the Gouderak scandal was breaking, for example, a government-commissioned report by three Rotterdam lawyers revealed that Uniser Holding, a waste disposal company which went bankrupt and whose directors were gaoled in 1981 for fraud and illegal dumping and sales of waste, operated with the cooperation of highly placed Dutch ministry officials and civil servants working at many different levels of responsibility.

To the dismay of many industrialists, the environmental pressure on their operations showed no signs of abating, despite the recession of the early 1980s. At the 1983 annual meeting of the German chemical company Hoechst, for example, it turned out that about 2,000 shares had been bought by members of the country's Greens and of several Frankfurt environmental groups. They took the podium as shareholders to demand that Hoechst should spend its total dividend of DM259 million on environmental protection, rather than paying it out as a dividend of DM 5.50 per share. Other shareholders, perhaps not surprisingly, were less enthusiastic.

Hoechst, in fact, was one of the companies which had been branded as 'pollution criminals' by a Rhine Tribunal organized by environmentalists from Switzerland, France, West Germany, Luxembourg and the Netherlands, all of which lie along the river's course. 'If you want photos developed,' one Dutch joke runs, 'throw them in the Rhine.' But the pollution of the river is no laughing matter for such countries as Holland which take a great deal of water from the Rhine for use in such applications as horticulture. Providing drinking water for some twenty million Europeans, the Rhine still contains nearly 2,000 chemicals. As well as Hoechst, the alliance of environmentalists accused the potash mines of Alsace and companies such as BASF, Bayer, Ciba-Geigy, Hoffman-La Roche, Rhône Poulenc and Sandoz of 'pollution crimes'.

One group that did not support the tribunal idea was Greenpeace, which argued that the facts are well known and that only direct action would convince industry that it cannot use rivers such as the Rhine as industrial sewers. Although the Environment Minister for the State of Hesse had recently accused two Hoechst subsidiaries of releasing such chemicals as chloroform (a suspected carcinogen), carbon tetrachloride (another suspected carcinogen) and trichloroethylene (a suspected mutagen) into the river Main, which flows into the Rhine, Greenpeace decided in 1980 to go for Bayer. They were perturbed to find that Bayer had been given permission by the Dutch Minister for Transport and Waterways to dump 550,000 tonnes of acid wastes a year in the sea not far from Scheveningen.

Those wastes, Greenpeace discovered, contained many carcinogens and were contaminated by very considerable quantities of chromium, lead, copper, zinc, cadmium and mercury. It also found that every working day barges sailed from Bayer's enormous production site at Leverkusen for Rotterdam, where their cargoes were offloaded into two coasters which, in turn, sailed two or three times a day to the dumping grounds. The Oslo Convention, Greenpeace knew, forbids the dumping at sea of many of these substances.

The Minister later instructed Bayer to carry out the dumping thirty kilometres further out to sea and to reduce the rate at which the wastes were discharged, to ensure better mixing. But Greenpeace was convinced Bayer was still acting illegally. So it began a blockade, using inflatable, motorized dinghies and trapping the two coasters in harbour. It issued a statement demanding that Bayer stop dumping wastes in the North Sea; that the Dutch government should explain why it was violating the Oslo and London Conventions; that any future permits should be issued only after ecological and toxicity tests had been carried out with the fauna and flora actually found at the dumping grounds in the North and Wadden Seas; and that any future dump site should be located well away from commercial fishing grounds and should be regularly monitored.

Bayer's initial response was to ask the authorities for permission to dump into the Rhine each year, after treatment, 250,000 tonnes of dilute acid, a practice it had been the first to stop in 1969. The company also stated that 4,000 jobs were at stake in the plants likely to be affected by the ban. Later, too, Bayer managed to end the blockade by threatening punitive damages against Greenpeace – but it did not leave matters there. First, it invited members of Greenpeace to immediate discussions with top management, including the managing director of the Leverkusen site, Professor Eberhard Weise. Second, it invited Greenpeace to send a small group of observers at a later date to see what the company was doing to overcome the acid problem.

Paradoxically, the company had been one of the most environmentally sensitive of all West Germany's chemical companies, featuring environmental protection in its annual reports and, indeed, in its corporate logo: a green linden leaf emblazoned with the motto 'Bayer research for a clean environment'. In 1980 alone, it pointed out, its capital expenditure on environmental protection had amounted to DM 165 million, while its environmental operating costs increased from DM 410 million to DM 485 million, compared with after-tax profits of DM 348 million.

Greenpeace had known nothing of this when it decided to tackle Bayer, believing it was a case of an ecological David versus a German Goliath, with little inkling that it was up against something which considered itself a Green Giant. Bayer was also taken aback, believing that its acid dumping in the North Sea was ecologically preferable to dumping the same wastes in the Rhine. And, to be fair, when Bayer took a small group including Dr Alan Pickaver of Greenpeace, Brian Price (pollution consultant to Friends of the Earth), and myself (as an independent observer with some knowledge of what other chemical companies had been able to achieve) around its various production sites, we were all impressed by the progress Bayer had been able to make in dealing with this highly complex problem. By the time we toured the sites, the company was recycling the equivalent of 122,000 tonnes of 20 per cent sulphuric acid each year.

Acid recycling, like many other forms of recycling, is a problem activity, the problem here being the corrosiveness of the various process streams. The recycled acid costs five or six times as much as acid produced from scratch, which hardly makes the exercise a commercial proposition. A much happier approach, and one which we saw in operation at Bayer's new production site at Brunsbuettel, involves the development and deployment of cleaner, low-waste technologies. Of five plants built in the first stage of construction at this vast 1,000-acre site, which is unlikely to be completely developed before the year 2020, two were recycling plants designed to bring waste materials back into the production process. By the time we got there, wet air oxidation and incineration plants were also in operation, detoxifying or destroying toxic wastes.

Clearly, in those industries which are continuing to invest in new sites and new technologies a great deal can be done to cut the output of pollutants per tonne of product manufactured. Indeed, I was responsible for a study, commissioned by the Department of the Environment's Central Directorate on Environmental Pollution, which concluded that current trends in the structure of the British economy and developments in the technologies likely to be deployed through the 1980s and 1990s were likely to help substantially in cutting many forms of pollution. Similar conclusions have emerged from studies in a number of countries, including the United States. In summary, the older, more environment-intensive industries have been falling apart, while the newer industries typically show a much higher return, in terms of value added, for each unit of pollution. Indeed some industries, such as the microelectronics industry, have tended themselves to be acutely sensitive to other people's pollution, which can contaminate and disrupt the delicate chip circuitry and other technologies with which they work.

That said, some of these newer industries have themselves run into major pollution problems. ITT Semiconductors, for example, was the source of a massive accidental leak of caustic soda which wiped out fish stocks in the river Cray in England. And, in the United States, Fairchild Camera & Instrument and Intel are among companies which have been pinpointed as pollution sources. Both are based in California's Silicon Valley and both reported leaks of toxic chemicals: 1,1,1-trichloroethane, a degreasing agent, in the case of Fairchild, and the far more toxic trichloroethylene in the case of Intel. Although there is limited evidence from animal studies suggesting that trichloroethylene is not teratogenic at levels up to 1,800 parts per million, it is known to cross the placenta readily, is possibly carcinogenic in mice, and there is some evidence that it may be a human mutagen.

When William Ruckelshaus took over the EPA for the second time, he stressed that 'we must now assume that life takes place in a minefield of risks from hundreds, perhaps thousands of substances'. Some of these, as we have seen, can cause cancer, birth defects or chromosomal damage. Accepting that 'many communities are gripped by something approaching panic' in the face of pollution problems, he said that governments can no longer assure their citizens that they will be protected from all risk. 'One thing we clearly need to do,' he said, 'is to ensure that our laws reflect these scientific realities. The administrator of the EPA should not be forced to represent that a margin of safety exists for a specific substance at a specific level of exposure where none can be scientifically valid.'

Ideally, governments would like to be able to set hard and fast thresholds for human exposure to chemical and other threats to health. They would like to be able to report that exposure to, say, 100 parts per million of chemical X is possibly dangerous, but 50 parts per million are unquestionably no threat to health. Unfortunately, as the relevant sciences have pressed forward, it has become increasingly obvious that many such thresholds are illusory: health effects can emerge, given suitable circumstances, at levels of exposure previously thought totally safe. This is partly because some of us are genetically predisposed to damage by certain chemicals and partly because many of the chemicals we manufacture, use and dispose of with such abandon are proving to be rather more insidiously harmful than had been suspected. For example, we may imagine that dumping a particular waste in the North Sea rather than the Rhine is ecologically preferable, and ecologically preferable it may be. But this does not mean that it is ecologically harmless, or that we will not at some later date discover some feedback loop in the ecosystem which has been causing unsuspected and detrimental ecological or human health effects.

Clearly, as Greenpeace suggested when tackling Bayer, we have got to know a great deal more about the ecological and human health implications of the chemicals we use. But before we turn to some of the tests now being developed to pinpoint possible chemical carcinogens, teratogens or mutagens, it is worth considering briefly the recent history of lead additives in petrol, which illustrates both the ways that presumed 'no-effect' thresholds can prove treacherous and the degree to which the question of relative risk brings politics into the pollution control equation.

Lead is among the most ubiquitous of pollutants, and it has also been repeatedly branded as a major threat to various aspects of human reproduction. It is a neurotoxin, affecting the brain and central nervous system. Children and the unborn are particularly vulnerable because their nervous systems, together with the protective membranes insulating their brains from their bloodstreams, are still developing.

If we were to compile a list of the peoples and populations which have been most exposed to lead through history, the Romans would emerge either in the top slot, or very close to it. When a Roman cemetery was excavated near Cirencester, which was the second largest Roman city in Britain, the 450 skeletons found were discovered to have up to ten times as much lead in their bones as does today's man or woman in the street. 'There are a great number of medical works which indicate that there were great pandemics of lead poisoning through the Roman empire,' said Dr H. A. Waldron of the London School of Hygiene and Tropical Medicine. Dr Waldron had carried out the research on the lead content of the bones and confirmed that the probable cause was the Romans' dietary habits. Lead was widely used in cooking implements and in water pipes. Worse, bad wine was sometimes improved by the simple expedient of adding lead. As we have seen (p. 55) the poisoning of the Roman reproductive system was aggravated when traditional injunctions against the drinking of wine by women were relaxed.

Even today we have a surprising quantity of lead piping still in use, although the main focus of public concern has been the health impact of lead in petrol. Lead from drinking water is nevertheless just as dangerous to children, indeed some researchers believe that children absorb more lead from water than from the air. An EEC Directive has committed member states to reducing the lead content of tapwater to a level below 100 milligrams per litre, but the cost of removing lead piping from the two million British houses where the water still delivers its daily dose of lead has been estimated at £1 billion. Given that householders would have to pay much of this bill, this option has tended to be seen as a political non-starter.

Meanwhile, however, Water Research Centre scientists have discovered that dosing the water with orthophosphoric acid can significantly cut the rate at which lead dissolves into tapwater – which raises the possibility that lead exposure could be cut in many areas without stripping out all the old pipework.

The exhaust pipe of the ordinary family car, however, has still tended to be seen as the most pernicious threat. The two main questions raised in the debate about lead in petrol through the early 1980s were these: Is there a 'safe' threshold level of exposure for such vulnerable groups as children? And how much of the lead burden they already carry can be attributed to lead in petrol?

The level of blood lead considered acceptable has been falling in many countries. In 1982, for example, the Department of the Environment told local councils around Britain that although levels of up to 35 milligrams per 100 millilitres of blood were acceptable, the environments of children found to have blood lead levels over 25 milligrams should be investigated. But new research results continued to flood in, some of them suggesting that lead in petrol was contributing considerably more to total lead burdens than most health experts had imagined. One such study was carried out by the EEC's Joint Research Centre at Ispra, Italy. Working with an oil company, Agip Petroli, and two producers of lead anti-knock additives, the Ethyl Corporation and the Società Italiana Additivi Carburanti, the Centre came up with results which its industrial collaborators must have found less than satisfying.

Instead of confirming earlier results suggesting that perhaps 10 per cent of our blood lead comes from petrol, the study found that at least 25 per cent could be attributed to this source in Turin. The experiment used lead from the Broken Hill mine in Australia, which contains a pair of radioactive isotopes identifying it as clearly as a set of fingerprints. This lead was added to 90 per cent of the petrol sold in the Turin area and a large sample of people was monitored to see how much of the tagged lead showed up in their blood.

Meanwhile, in the United States, a survey of blood lead levels in 27,800 people found there had been an average decrease of 37 per cent in those blood lead levels between 1976 and 1980. The only explanation the researchers could come up with was that this drop reflected the impact of the country's policy of phasing out lead in petrol from 1974. Over the same period, the amount of lead used in petrol fell by 50 per cent. The reason behind the policy decision, or at least the primary reason, was that the lead was poisoning the catalysts used on new cars to eliminate other forms of air pollution. But then health considerations came to the fore, encouraging the EPA to resist pressure from the White House to slow up on lead controls.

The political dimension of the lead debate is perhaps best illustrated by the experience in Britain, where the government was persuaded by mounting scientific evidence to announce that from 1985 the maximum amount of lead in petrol would be reduced from 0.4 to 0.15 grams per litre. Some environmentalists saw this as a victory, and the government, the oil industry and the motor manufacturers hoped that that would be that. Far from it.

The launch of the Campaign for Lead-Free Air (CLEAR) early in 1982 heralded the next stage of the battle. An unlikely alliance between a consummate campaigner and a millionaire who made his money by advising clients on tax avoidance transformed the picture and forced a major cave-in on the part of the government and the oil companies. Godfrey Bradman, who backed CLEAR with £100,000 from his own pocket, had become so worried that lead emissions were damaging the health of his daughters that he had moved out of London. The other side of the alliance was Des Wilson, who had founded Shelter in 1966 to focus attention on the plight of Britain's homeless. Although initially unsure whether he wanted to develop another single-issue campaign, Wilson was angered by the refusal of the oil companies to meet him to discuss the lead controversy. 'That was their big mistake,' he said later. 'They made me angry at being brushed off – and I don't brush off easily.'

Soon an absolute godsend dropped into his lap, by courtesy of an unnamed Whitehall 'mole'. This was a letter written by the government's own chief medical officer, Sir Henry Yellowlees. Admitting that he was taking an 'unusual step', Sir Henry wrote

to Sir James Hamilton, Permanent Secretary at the Department of
Education and Science, suggesting that a great deal had changed
since the publication of the 1980 Lawther Report on the effects of
low levels of lead on children's intelligence, learning ability and
behaviour. The working party, chaired by Professor Pat Lawther,
had remained unconvinced about the threat posed by low levels
of lead, although it accepted that somewhat higher levels could
give cause for concern. Because of the general uncertainties involved, however, the working party recommended that the
government should take a number of steps to reduce population
exposure to the metal.

'There is no doubt,' Sir Henry noted in his letter, 'that the
simplest and quickest way of reducing general population exposure
to lead is by reducing sharply or by entirely eliminating lead
in petrol.' He continued to say that 'there is a strong likelihood
that lead in petrol is permanently reducing the IQ of many
of our children. Although the reduction amounts to only a few
percentage points, some hundreds of thousands of children are
affected.'

The government was shaken by the publication of the letter, but
decided to hang on until the Royal Commission on Environmental
Pollution published its own report on lead. When the Royal Commission did so, early in 1983, it reported that 'the average blood
lead concentration in the population is about one quarter of that
at which symptoms of frank poisoning may occasionally occur. We
find this disturbing.' It also pointed out that 'we do not know of
any other toxic substance which is both so widely distributed in
human and animal populations and present at concentrations
greater than even one tenth of those at which frank symptoms may
occur. We consider this reason enough to seek to reduce the
exposure of the general population to lead.'   The scale of lead use
in a country like Britain is indicated by the fact that at that time
about 274.000 tonnes a year were being used, compared with
strikingly lower levels for other heavy metals such as cadmium
(1,350 tonnes) and mercury (510 tonnes). Announcing his
decision to press for an EEC-wide ban on lead in petrol, the Secretary of State for the Environment, Mr Tom King, called attention
to his rapid response to the Commission's report. But there were
those who felt he was taking slight liberties with the facts. For,
while the report presented some research results in a slightly
different light, there was nothing in it which had not been known

in May 1981, when the government opted for a reduction of lead in petrol rather than an outright ban.

Even more strangely, the Commission failed to come down on either side of the fence as far as CLEAR's central argument was concerned. Does lead affect children's intelligence at low levels of exposure? 'The accumulated evidence,' the Commission suggested, 'may indicate a causal association between the body burden of lead and psychometric indices, or the effects of confounding factors, or both. On present evidence we do not consider it possible to distinguish between these possibilities.'

Nothing, in short, had really changed. But *The Times* summed up the reaction in a leader entitled 'Good Riddance to Lead'. 'Where the science of the subject may admit doubt,' it said, 'the politics of the subject knows no such hesitation. It is now past the point where the onus of proof shifts from those who challenge current practices to those who would defend them. It is no longer necessary to show that a thick urban environment exposes children to the risks considered: it is necessary to show that it does not. And the second can be done no more conclusively than the first. The children, not the lead, get the benefit of the doubt; and when the matter is put like that, who would dare to dispute it?'

Some people in the oil industry continued to dispute it, but the government knew an election was imminent. To promise lead-free petrol by 1990, and perhaps even by 1987, seemed an acceptable political price to pay for peace and quiet on the environmental front.

The lead controversy illustrates a fact of modern life: we are increasingly having to make decisions about environmental and health issues which will have enormous implications for important sectors of industry – and we are having to do so on the basis of evidence which can be interpreted in a variety of ways. In cases where the human reproductive system is threatened, it is clearly possible in a democracy to shift entrenched attitudes and to dislodge powerful vested interests from prepared positions. But much of the disputed evidence is being generated by test systems which are themselves the subject of controversy. We now turn to look at some of these test systems – and at some of the uncertainties that surround them.

CHAPTER SEVEN

TESTING TIMES

The news could hardly have been worse. Given that the purpose of testing the toxicity of chemical and pharmaceutical products is to reassure both the public and the regulatory authorities that they are safe, the news that a major toxicity testing company had not only been producing flawed data but had on occasion actively faked its results came as something of a body-blow to the testing industry and to industries which use its testing facilities.

When a US court finally handed down judgements on three former officials of Industrial Bio-Test Laboratories, Inc. (IBT), it did so on eight counts of falsifying laboratory data. The products involved were: Nemacur and Sencor, pesticides made by Chemagro Corporation, a division of Mobay Chemical Corporation of Pittsburgh; Naprosyn, an arthritic drug made by Syntex Corporation of Palo Alto, California; and trichlorocarbanilide, an anti-bacterial agent used in many soaps. All these products were later re-tested by other laboratories and found to be safe, but these charges were simply the tip of an iceberg. IBT had been under investigation since 1976, seven years before the judgements were announced. Some months previously, the Environmental Protection Agency had published a final review of 801 health studies which IBT had carried out. Of the 594 studies of pesticides, for example, 140 were judged invalid.

The Agency promptly gave the manufacturers of nineteen of these pesticides a period of three months in which to complete replacement tests, under threat of suspension if they failed to do so. The Canadian authorities reviewed forty-three pesticides whose clearances had been based on IBT tests, and promptly banned three of them: cyprazine, chlorobromuron and Gardall. Another twenty-three products were required to carry labels warning users that the product's safety was now open to question. Four of the pesticides which the EPA had ordered re-tested immediately were in fairly common use in Britain at the time: chlorobromuron, methazol, phenthoate and sodium chlorate. However, their safety had been reviewed some years earlier when it was first learned that some of the IBT tests might be suspect.

Most of these products clearly had a history of years of safe use by the time the IBT scandal broke and they found themselves once again on the suspect list. None the less, the damage caused went a great deal beyond these particular products, however valuable their various markets may have been. The public, its politicians and the regulatory authorities were left with a whole clutch of question marks, with some of the evidence given in court indicating that IBT had on occasion been persuaded by some of its major corporate clients to give its stamp of approval to products whose toxicity was already in doubt.

Monsanto, Olin and FMC were three former IBT clients who found themselves enmired in the scandal. A federal report filed in court claimed that these three corporations knowingly submitted flawed data to the EPA in support of a widely used swimming pool chlorinator, a product which some suspected to be a cause of kidney and bladder problems. Other documents filed alleged that IBT's president, sixty-five-year-old Dr Joseph Calandra, who was not in court along with his aides because he had been hospitalized for major heart surgery, had bowed to pressure from Monsanto on another of its products, the sugar-cane herbicide butachlor, which the company planned to market under the trade name Machete. Calandra, it was alleged, had agreed to soften IBT's assessment from 'mildly tumorigenic' to 'does not appear to be carcinogenic'.

The particular concern as far as the pool chlorinator was concerned was the ingredient monosodium cyanurate, which earlier studies had shown to cause serious kidney problems in test animals. In fact, it was charged, one of IBT's studies had to be revised when, over a period of three months, an entire test animal group was wiped out by kidney and bladder problems which appeared to be associated with monosodium cyanurate. Monsanto, the federal report claimed, had experienced similar problems with its own in-house testing. The investigators said that the three companies had disregarded these problems in their attempts to get their products to market. 'There were indications,' they suggested, 'that the kidney problems were deliberately overlooked in the conduct of the study, in spite of the client's awareness of the problems.'

Not surprisingly, Monsanto and the other companies charged vigorously denied the accusations. 'We deny Monsanto would knowingly submit any fraudulent data,' the company counter-attacked. But the publication of the charges inevitably raised larger questions in the public's mind. Even if IBT and its clients were given the benefit of the doubt and it was accepted that absolutely no falsification had occurred, which would be unduly generous in the face of the evidence, there is the much broader question of whether the results that such companies routinely submit to the regulatory authorities actually mean what they hope they mean.

Even industrial scientists have complained about the inaccuracy of some current toxicity tests. One, Dr David Salsburg of Pfizer Laboratories in Connecticut, has argued that tests used to assess the carcinogenicity of drugs and chemicals are about as accurate as flipping a coin would be, and he did the research to support his argument. He examined published data on 170 chemical compounds which had been tested on rodents by the National Cancer Institute. He also reviewed the literature on those chemicals known to cause human cancers – and found that of nineteen known carcinogens, only seven had been shown to cause cancer when fed to rodents. On this basis, flipping a coin might even be a better bet.

The basic test method he was interested in has become an industry standard. It involves feeding very high doses of particular chemicals to mice or rats. Once the animals have died, or have been killed, the toxicologists compare the rate and pattern of tumour formation in the animals which were dosed and in control groups of animals which were not. Dr Salsburg is a statistician, so he applied a number of increasingly rigorous statistical tests to this test method, to see how often it would produce false negatives (failing to identify known carcinogens) or false positives (incriminating an innocuous substance). 'We have an assay test,' he concluded, 'that may be wrong 50 per cent of the time.'

Again, there were protests. The deputy director of the US

National Toxicology Programme claimed that Salsburg's critique contained 'distortions and errors'. Salsburg had pointed out that the National Cancer Institute had concluded that half of the substances it had studied were carcinogens, but it was retorted that the Institute picks substances for testing which are already suspected of posing a risk to health.

Such scientific differences of opinion are not the only problems that today's toxicologists have to face. 'We will run up against difficulties,' Lammot du Pont had warned at the dedication of the E. I. du Pont de Nemours & Co., Inc. Haskell Laboratory as long ago as 1935. 'For instance, the operating department will want to know "why the laboratory doesn't produce something". The sales department will want to know "why the laboratory works up data that might make our customers believe our products are unsafe". But,' he concluded, 'we are embarked on our campaign with determination and it is only a question of time before the world recognizes that a very constructive thing has been done.'

Even he might have been surprised to find out how long it has taken some of Du Pont's competitors to get around to this view. Du Pont, like many of the companies which moved into toxicology at an early stage, had its reasons for doing so. Founded in 1802 to manufacture explosives, it soon hit problems. An explosion in 1818 killed forty employees. The company's founder, Eleuthère Irénée du Pont, assumed responsibility for the establishment and enforcement of safe practices. In the early days of capitalism, this might have been simply a ruse to keep the whole area under wraps, but in Du Pont this early commitment by top management gave considerable momentum to the question of employee safety.

The company maintains that all injuries can be prevented, and by 1978 it was able to report that there had been only one disabling accident for each four million man-hours worked in its factories, one-fiftieth of the rate for all industry and one-sixteenth of the rate reported for the US chemical industry as a whole. But Du Pont's goal had never been zero risks. It accepts that there will always be some element of risk in any industrial operation.

The hazards facing the company's employees had multiplied when it was transformed from an explosives manufacturer into a diversified chemical manufacturer after the First World War. As Du Pont itself recalls, 'workers exposed to carbon disulfide cellophane and rayon were showing toxic effects. Those making tetraethyl lead, the gasoline antiknock additive, faced the danger of lead poisoning. And it was discovered in the early 1930s that beta-napthylamine, an intermediate used in the making of coal tar dyes, was related to an unusually high incidence of employee bladder tumors.' The establishment of the Haskell Laboratory was part of the company's response.

By the early 1980s Haskell was employing over 200 people, a fifth of whom had doctorates covering such disciplines as molecular biology and microbiology, chemistry and biochemistry, aquatic toxicology, biostatistics and pathology. Each year it was testing about 700 chemical substances for possible toxic effects and maintaining a test animal population of about 10,000, 95 per cent of which were rodents. Sometimes it recommended that a material be dropped, as when it tested a brominated biphenyl which Du Pont had found to be highly effective in protecting synthetic fibres against fire.

Like the sixteenth-century scientist Paracelsus, Du Pont has felt it prudent to proceed on the assumption that 'all things are poisons. Only the dose decides that a thing is not poisonous.' Haskell's task is therefore to find an acceptable exposure level for chemicals used in Du Pont factories and contained in its products. 'The classic procedure,' it says, 'is to expose laboratory animals to test compounds, to identify clinical signs that may be produced, to find the dose-response relationship, and to project the findings to human situations.'

The company admits that acute hazards, which cause injury or illness through an accident or once-off exposure, remain a stubborn problem, while it points out that 'the dimensions of chronic hazard problems are only just coming to light'. These hazards, it stresses, 'are more subtle, more insidious and more complex than most dangers previously encountered in the workplace'.

By 1980, Du Pont had classified as possible animal or human carcinogens thirty-six chemicals, ranging from by-products present in very small amounts to chemicals such as carbon tetrachloride which are intermediates for high-volume products. One such classified compound was the solvent used in making 'Kevlar' aramid fibre. As Du Pont explains, 'in the case of this material, hexamethylphosphoramide (HMPA), there had been no prior studies indicating that it was a carcinogen before Du Pont began its tests. When long-term animal tests showed it to be carcinogenic, Du Pont notified employees, federal and state agencies, and scientific journals. Employee exposures were reduced to 0.5 parts per billion.'

One of Du Pont's recent epidemiological studies focused on employees potentially exposed to acrylonitrile at one of its plants. The study showed that employees first exposed to acrylonitrile in the early 1950s were more likely to develop cancer than the average company employee, raising the suspicion that it might be a human carcinogen. Interestingly, when the Guy's Hospital Medical School team reviewed the literature on acrylonitrile, whose applications have ranged from the manufacture of acrylic fibre to its use as a pesticide fumigant for stored grain, it found that Du Pont was not alone in its concern. The evidence, however, proved patchy. It found that acrylonitrile is carcinogenic in rats, but it found no data on any transplacental carcinogenicity. It is mutagenic in bacteria, with activation, and there is some evidence to suggest that it can be embryotoxic and teratogenic in rats at doses which are also toxic to the mother rat, but the team found no data on fertility effects.

Du Pont's study at its Camden plant took several years to complete, with 1,350 employees involved, many of whom had left the company and had to be traced through Social Security files and other means. Employee exposures were cut from 20 parts per million to 2 parts per million, a level later adopted by the US Occupational Safety and Health Administration as its permissible workplace exposure level. Du Pont, however, remained uncertain as to whether acrylonitrile is a carcinogen, arguing that only further epidemiological research would resolve the matter.

The toxicity testing boom has produced a rapid growth in the number and turnover of privately owned contract toxicity research laboratories. Among the first of these was Food and Drug Research Laboratories, launched shortly after the First World War, but it was not until after the Second World War that toxicity testing really began to take off. Industrial Bio-Test dated from this period, as do the toxicity testing activities of other well-known names such as Arthur D. Little, Battelle, Hazelton, Stamford Research and Woodward Labs, all in the USA. In the UK, Alastair Worden founded his Nutritional Research Unit, subsequently re-named the Huntingdon Research Centre.

There were problems, of course. Arthur D. Little tried to break into the European market with an offshoot in Scotland. The attempt was unsuccessful, and the activity was acquired by members of the company's staff and by other interests and now operates as Inveresk Research International. Stanford Research also tried to develop a European activity, but the venture did not go as well as expected. Huntingdon tried to break into the US market by establishing a laboratory there, but were later forced to cut back their presence there.

The 1960s saw a plethora of new companies, including American ventures (Biodynamics, Bionetics, Bioresearch, IRDC and Leberco) and European ventures (including one established by TNO, the government-controlled Dutch laboratory). During the 1970s the number of new, traditionally based private laboratory formations fell, with Life Science Research, a sister venture to Biodynamics, falling into this category. Most of the new starts resulted from collaboration between government and industry, with examples emerging in such countries as France, Italy and Japan. Then, in the late 1970s, the rate of new company formations picked up again, with the emergence of companies such as Toxicol in Britain and at least ten significant new competitors in the USA.

Before discussing some of the specific tests which have been developed to pinpoint substances which may act as carcinogens, teratogens or mutagens, we can get a much better idea of the business environment in which such concerns operate by focusing on one of them: Life Science Research (LSR). 'You could say we were no longer happy working in the Huntingdon environment,' says Dr Ken Harper, now director of LSR, but previously director-general of the Huntingdon Research Centre. The idea of setting up a new laboratory, he says, 'came very, very suddenly. It wasn't pre-planned. Things came to a head.'

When LSR first opened its doors in 1972, Dr Harper recalls, 'We did not have a single client.' However, by word-of-mouth and personal contacts the news got around. Indeed, the company had put together a five-year business plan when looking for backing, and now found that it had reached its revenue target for its fifth year of operation by the end of its first year. 'Almost fortuitously,' Dr Harper observes, 'we chose the right moment. It wasn't through any detailed study of the business environment at the time. It happened to coincide with an explosion in toxicology.'

LSR competed with Industrial Bio-Test in Japan, says Dr Harper, 'and we were always amazed by their low prices. We had no reason to suspect foul play: they had a fairly good reputation and dated back to the 1950s.' Scandals such as that which broke around

Industrial Bio-Test have ensured that the contract research sector operates under increasingly tight scrutiny. 'It's a question of Big Brother's watching,' Dr Harper explains, 'and someone's watching Big Brother.' LSR's clients closely monitor what is going on, as do the public sector agencies such as the Department of Health and Social Security and the Health Safety Executive. In addition, shortly before I visited them, LSR had been given a thorough going over by the Japanese, with the Japanese market representing a significant element in the company's operations.

Whether they work in industrial, government or contract laboratories, today's toxicologists have to adopt 'good laboratory practice' which, Dr Harper says, 'has been a great equalizer. It has meant that there has been no place for the cut-price laboratory. Everyone now has to meet certain minimum standards.' These new guidelines, he believes, are 'a very useful management tool. People now have to work within very strict operating limits. Even the prima donna scientist is now accountable.' Dr Colin Roberts, another LSR director who previously worked with Huntingdon, points out that their introduction probably made relatively little difference to the better-run laboratories. 'The fact that you're now writing in ink rather than in pencil doesn't materially affect your findings,' he says, but he accepts that the guidelines have forced many companies to put their toxicity testing activities on a much more professional footing.

The cost of these improvements has not been insignificant. Good laboratory practice has resulted in higher prices throughout the industry. LSR reckon that it has increased this element of their charges from less than 40 per cent five years ago to about 60 per cent today. Such increases proved a particular problem during the recession of the early 1980s. 'It used to be the case that in times of recession we would prosper,' says Dr Harper, 'since industry cut back on its in-house research. But the present recession has cut so deeply that even we have been affected.'

The outlook in the new drugs area is far from bleak, however. 'There are an amazing number of new products coming along,' Dr Harper observes. 'Each company seems to have a fistful of molecules it wants to develop. They've taken the lid off spending and they're coming through to us for the next stage in their development. These are not me-too products. They are tending to be novel molecules. Even Japan has some novel molecules,' he says. 'You can no longer say that they are just copying.'

One of the healthiest parts of LSR's business has been its reproductive toxicity testing. Dr John Tesh, who runs this side of the company's operations, calculates that about 40 per cent of their work in this area focuses on agro-chemicals and 60 per cent on drugs, with little change in these proportions over recent years. He agrees that major changes are going on in the drug industry, with a growing requirement for tests of a drug's potential for causing behavioural aberrations beyond birth in test animals (or humans) exposed in the womb.

'Since thalidomide and the full realization of the effects that drugs and other agents may have on the developing foetus,' Dr Tesh says, 'a great deal of effort has been expended upon establishing procedures to safeguard the early stages of pregnancy, but relatively little towards the later stages. Previously,' he points out, 'guidelines for drug safety assessment contained very brief suggestions concerning post-natal investigation of offspring. However, relatively recently there has been a growing concern amongst workers in the field of reproductive toxicology that the areas of late gestation and early post-natal life should be examined in greater detail.'

If such problems emerge, today's pharmaceutical and chemical producers may well find themselves open to the same challenge that faced Chemie Grünenthal after thalidomide's side-effects surfaced. 'In the ten years preceding the appearance of thalidomide, that is by 1959,' charged Professor John B. Thiersch, director of the Institute of Biological Research and Professor of Clinical Pharmacology at the University of Seattle, 'not less than twenty-five compounds were shown by various investigators, ranging from Japan to the United States, to England and France, to affect the foetus *in utero*, either killing foetuses or inducing malformations.' But could Chemie Grünenthal have picked up these specific problems with existing test methods? 'The answer,' the internationally known teratologist Professor Walter Landauer said in his evidence, 'must be emphatically in the affirmative.'

The available methods, Professor Thiersch explained, 'consisted of obtaining the foetuses from the uterus of pregnant animals or newborns, inspecting them, measuring them, fixing them in various fixatives, cutting the foetuses in serial sections for microscopic studies, clearing and staining their skeletons with oil of wintergreen, alizarine and methylene blue. In other instances, X-ray photos were taken to study the malformation of the skeleton.'

In conclusion, he said, 'One has to say that the methods used later in an attempt to define the action of thalidomide on the embryo were well established before 1959.'

The underlying science has made major strides since, of course, and the effectiveness of our checkpoints for identifying teratogens has improved enormously. 'If all the products that we have seen over the last twenty years had gone to market,' Dr Tesh points out, 'there would have been quite a number of teratogens.'

Others saw a different message to the thalidomide saga. 'It is a piece of history now documented repeatedly how, following thali-domide, more and more statutory checks were built into the opera-tions of the pharmaceutical industry,' says Dr Sam Shuster, Pro-fessor of Dermatology at the University of Newcastle upon Tyne, 'all in the flawed belief that we could prevent more disaster by testing. The real message of thalidomide was never heard: it is that ill-effects of drugs are inevitable and that social acceptance of them is the real price of drugs.'

This surely overstates the case, but the regularity with which new drugs that have gone through the full battery of current tests continue to produce unexpected side-effects underscores the fact that no one can ever guarantee that a drug, an industrial chemical or a crop protection product is safe, even if used according to the manufacturer's instructions. The other side of the coin has been an astonishing rise in the cost of testing such drugs and chemicals. Between 1969 and 1978, the cost of developing a new drug in Britain almost quadrupled in real terms, from £15 million in 1969 to about £58 million in 1978. Five years later, the cost was estimated to be between £50 million and £100 million over ten years, and a similar trend has been seen in the costs of testing crop protection chemicals.

'If you sat down and wrote out what you wanted from a com-pound,' I was told by Dr John Leahey, a senior research officer at ICI's Jealott's Hill Research Station, 'that compound was Fusillade. It was a dream compound, the first on which I have worked where everywhere you looked it was the way you wanted it.' But that new herbicide, first marketed in 1982, was simply the luck of the draw at work: eventually something must fit the bill in every respect. Most compounds which prove to have some activity which could be of value in the crop protection business also prove to have at least some environmental or health side-effects, which need to be carefully evaluated both in the laboratory and in field tests.

Even with a product like its pirimicarb aphicide, marketed as Aphox and Rapid, ICI had a fairly tough time persuading both regulators and potential customers of the product's extraordinary selectivity. 'It took a lot of testing to convince people that it is safe to spray an insecticide on a flowering crop where bees are present,' Dr Leahey recalled. 'But it is safe. In fact it is so safe that it is an ideal chemical for use in integrated pest control programmes.'

Shell Chemical were making similar claims on behalf of their new insecticide, alphamethrin, marketed as Fastac, at the same time. Descended from the highly successful synthetic pyrethroid family of insecticides, Fastac was described by Shell as the 'best insecticide we have ever made'. The company had spent more than £1 million on ecological tests to back up its claim that Fastac was unusually safe in the environment. 'To maintain our lead in the extremely competitive insecticides market, where in some countries spraying costs per hectare have been halved in real terms over the last five years,' said Neville Craig, project coordinator for Fastac, 'we have had to go one step further.' Fastac proved to have a high chemical activity, which means that less is used and thus less escapes into the environment, and it also proved to be effective against a broad range of pests, including stalk borers, bollworms, weevils and beetles. Because it kills these pests at twenty to a hundred times lower dose than widely used commodity agro-chemicals, Fastac came out as comparable in cost with methyl parathion which, unlike Fastac, kills bees.

Clearly, these are the sort of products which would convince even some of the hard-nosed critics who worried Lammot du Pont when he opened the Haskell Laboratory, but ICI's figures suggest that Shell's £1 million figure should be considered as a minimum cost for the ecological studies now required. When I first visited the environmental sciences group at Jealott's Hill, it employed around a hundred people, with about twenty-five involved in ecological studies, fifty involved in metabolism and residue studies, and twenty-five following through on product registration. The group's activities were also supported by considerable numbers of people working at the company's Central Toxicology Laboratory and at its Brixham Laboratory. The average cost of taking a new pesticide from discovery to large-scale manufacture, according to ICI, had increased from about £1.5 million in 1965 to about £3 million in 1970. But by the time I first visited Jealott's Hill, in 1979, that figure had reached £15 million – with toxicological, ecological and environmental testing accounting for an average £3 million and taking seven years to complete. In fact, this element of product costs had been growing at about 30 per cent a year.

Today's new pesticides are probably subjected to more intensive environmental research than any other industrial product, which would have pleased Rachel Carson. Indeed, the financial risks involved in developing a new pesticide, or any other comparable chemical product, are very considerable. As Dr Green of ICI's Mond Division has put it, 'about 12,000 compounds on average have to be synthesized and screened to obtain one commercial product. Many of those which fail do so at a late stage in development, when a considerable amount of money has already been spent on them.' And, as another ICI executive stressed in 1979, 'our toxicology staff has increased from 200 to 300 over three years – where's the cut-off point? Where do we stop?'

Equally, where does a company like ICI start with its testing of a new crop protection chemical? In the early years of pesticide testing, the company's chemists and biologists look for answers to a whole range of questions. Is the product toxic to plants, insects and other animals – apart from those it is designed to kill? Is the product absorbed by plants and, if so, how does it behave once it is inside a plant? Does the product evaporate into the atmosphere or wash off into the soil? Does it accumulate, as the organo-chlorines did, in soil, birds or fish? As it breaks down in the environment, what are its breakdown products – and what happens to them? How soon after treatment is it safe to harvest the crop? Will there be harmful chemical residues in crops eaten by man or by animals? And so on down the spectrum of uncertainty.

Wherever possible, and for obvious reasons, the group prefers to carry out its tests in miniature, as in its bio-accumulation experiments, which are carried out in model ecosystems. One model ecosystem used by ICI consisted of an aquarium tank, with a bank of sand at one end and a pool of water at the other. Cabbages were grown in the sand and treated with a pesticide, whose molecules had been labelled with a radioactive atom (usually carbon-14, or ^{14}C). Caterpillars of the moth *Arctia caja* were then introduced to eat the cabbages, and some of them were later analysed for chemical residues. The remainder were drowned in the water and the decay products of their bodies eaten by small animals such as the protozoa, water fleas (*Daphnia*) and mosquito larvae (*Aedes aegyptii*).

Some of these, in turn, were analysed for residues. Finally, small fish were introduced to feed on the remaining *Daphnia* and mosquito larvae. The fish, as the final link in the food chain, were also analysed for residues.

And that is the chain in its simplest form. Other organisms, such as algae and snails, can be added for further studies. The next stages in the environmental screening of a new pesticide involve field trials on progressively larger plots of land. One of the major problems involved is that of sampling the species likely to be affected by incidental exposure, or by soil disturbance. ICI uses a range of sampling techniques, including pitfall traps (small plastic cups containing a preservative, embedded in the ground) and suction sampling – using what amounts to a large vacuum cleaner to suck organisms out of vegetation and into a collection bag.

The ecological testing of a new pesticide is designed to assess its effects on soils and soil micro-organisms, on predators and parasites of pests, on honeybees and other pollinators, on birds and mammals, and on the aquatic environment. One gram of soil can contain hundreds of millions of micro-organisms and there are ten thousand million grams of soil in one hectare of land to a depth of one metre. And one hectare of land can support more than a million earthworms, together with millions of other animals such as mites, springtails, millipedes, centipedes, woodlice, fly larvae, beetles and ants. Any predators and parasites of pests are important, with the growing recognition that integrated pest management must be the long-term goal, combining chemical and biological control methods. With this new emphasis, even if it is as yet embryonic, on the farmer's natural allies, new pesticides are screened for any effects on such insects as ladybirds, parasitic wasps and lacewings.

The economic importance of bees, particularly in crop pollination, has ensured that their health has become a major concern. Birds are also clearly at risk, largely because the preferred method of pesticide application is often seed dressing. ICI carries out extensive field trials in which it maps bird territories on experimental plots of up to fifty hectares. Any changes in the number or extent of these territories, or in the breeding success of the birds, are analysed, as are the tissues of a sample of the birds in the area. Laboratory tests and field trials are also used to investigate the effects of pesticides on mammalian wildlife and on farm and domesticated animals. Aquatic ecosystems are particularly sensitive to chemical pollution, so extensive aquatic toxicology tests are carried out both at Jealott's Hill and at the Brixham Laboratory. In the later stages of product development, these involve spraying and monitoring experimental ponds, lakes and streams.

The change that struck me most forcefully when I visited Jealott's Hill while in the final stages of writing this book was the enormously increased use of computers. Staff numbers were somewhat down on the 1979 levels, but the use of computers had been growing at an annual rate of something like 30 per cent. 'The way we are doing things is certainly the biggest change,' agreed research director Dr Peter Doyle, 'rather than what we are doing.' This trend, he said, coupled with the adoption of good laboratory practice and the new quality assurance methods, had brought 'astonishing changes'.

But, despite the often infernally complicated nature of the work which research units like Jealott's Hill carry out, the problems they face can sometimes look relatively uncomplicated when compared with those facing toxicologists who try to assess the implications of human exposure to a particular chemical.

Even if it is possible to calculate how many people have been exposed to the chemical, or are likely to be exposed to it, there are at least seven major steps before toxicologists can start human studies proper. Each of the various pieces of legislation covering ecological and toxicity testing tends to specify a different list of information requirements and a different array of tests, although the efforts of the Commission of the European Communities and the OECD have achieved a considerable degree of harmony in their members' regulatory requirements.

The first thing we need to know is what sort of chemical we are actually dealing with. We need to know its structure, the formulation of the product in which it will appear, the sort of processing it will undergo and its ultimate purity. It is often possible to suspect that a particular substance may be toxic simply because its chemical structure and properties are similar to those of known problem chemicals. The purity of the chemical is also vitally important, since an impure chemical may well act in a very different way than when in its pure form.

Chemical products likely to be subjected to toxicity testing include food additives and contaminants; cosmetics and toiletries;

household products and other consumer products, including some industrial chemicals; chemicals used in the formulation of medicines; and environmental pollutants. Clearly, absolute safety can never be guaranteed for any product, no matter how rigorous the test system. We are all genetically different from one another, responding in different ways to particular chemical threats, but even if we were all the same the impact of a chemical would depend on such factors as dosage, the physical state of those exposed, the other chemicals present at the time, and so on. Typically, too, estimates of risk and of the likely effects are based on animal and other laboratory tests which are far less certain than human studies would be.

Once a chemical is in use, it may prove to have an unfortunate effect on groups of people who, for one reason or another, are particularly susceptible. They may be genetically abnormal. They may be on special diets, or they may drink alcohol or smoke – all of which can affect an individual's response to chemicals. They may be elderly, with a number of age-related changes in our metabolism affecting the extent to which we are able to cope with such challenges. Or they may be foetuses, infants or children. Foetuses, as we have seen, may be vulnerable either because the chemical affects the mother or because it crosses the placenta, affecting the foetus directly. Infants and children tend to have a different range of detoxifying enzymes from adults, often lacking particular enzymes, which makes them particularly susceptible to such toxins, some of which may be excreted (and even concentrated) in the mother's milk.

The second major step in the vetting of a chemical involves the conduct of acute toxicity and 'target organ' studies. It is clearly vitally important that we know both the acute toxicity of a chemical and the organs in the human body which it is likely to affect or damage. Enormous controversy has surrounded the use of the LD_{50} test. The test involves feeding experimental animals with the chemical to be tested, or otherwise exposing them to it, to see at what level of exposure half the animals will be killed. Chemicals tend to be tested at a number of different dose levels, including a dose well above the point at which people are likely to suffer damage. It is also common to use two different animal species and to expose the experimental animals to the chemical by a number of different routes.

Toxicologists using the LD_{50} test are typically required to report any changes in the health and behaviour of the animals, particularly during the first twenty-four hours after they have been exposed to the chemical. They also note the number and timing of any deaths and describe what was found during post-mortems carried out on the experimental casualties and on survivors 'sacrificed' at the end of the experiment.

Even if none of the animals actually keels over and dies, it cannot be assumed that they have not suffered toxic effects. These tests are essentially short-term, lasting at most thirty days, whereas some of the repeated-dose tests we shall describe later may last three months, a year or, in some cases, even a number of years. Before deciding that such long-term studies are needed, it may make sense to establish which of the test animal's organs are being damaged by the chemical. In such 'target organ' studies, animals are dosed with the chemical for two to four weeks. The rat is usually picked for these studies, although if there are known to be wide differences between the response of the various species of test animals, a number of different species may be used. Such research clearly helps pinpoint a number of effects which may only emerge with cumulative doses, and it can also help establish so-called 'no-adverse-effect-levels' (NELs) – which legislators like to have to hand when setting exposure levels.

The third step centres on studies of the ways in which the metabolisms of experimental animals and people handle the chemical. Basically we want to know how much of the chemical is absorbed, how long it remains active in the bloodstream, where it goes and what it does when it gets there. Ideally, of course, the tests should be carried out in a species which handles the chemical in very much the same way as we do, but in practice this can be difficult. The preferred test animals in long-term research tend to be the rat, mouse and hamster, but the metabolism of different species can operate in very different ways and, even where they are fairly similar, they may produce very different 'minor metabolites', which are often found to be of considerable significance.

After it has been absorbed, from the gut or elsewhere, the target chemical may be distributed to various parts of the body. The toxicologist needs to know where it goes, how long it takes to get there, what happens to it along the way, and in what state it arrives at the target organ or site of interest. It is important to pin down the various ways in which the chemical and its breakdown products are excreted from the body, with excretion rates and routes often varying depending on the way in which the chemical itself is first administered.

If a chemical is excreted unchanged, then the problem may prove to be a relatively simple one, although this is by no means guaranteed. If, on the other hand, the chemical is broken down into a shower of metabolites, then it may be necessary to track each of them back 'upstream' in the metabolic process, to see where they were formed and what parts of the body they then passed through before being excreted.

One problem which needs to be constantly borne in mind is that the gut's bacterial enzymes may play an important role in forming and breaking down such metabolites, but these enzymes may vary from person to person. Age is an important factor here, of course, but so are the individual's genetic make-up and diet. A vegetarian, for example, may have a very different range of gut flora to that which flourishes in a non-vegetarian. Someone who regularly drinks alcohol may have a very different flora from that found in a teetotaller.

It may be necessary to test the chemical and some of its metabolites in a range of the digestive and other fluids found in the body, using *in vitro* methods involving mixing and analysing the chemical and fluids in a test-tube or flask. If a chemical is likely to be taken through the mouth, for example, it makes sense to test its stability in gastric or pancreatic juices. It may also be illuminating to study the metabolism of the chemical or of some of its metabolites by liver enzymes, to see if any short-lived substances are formed which potentially cause problems. This sort of research is likely to be more difficult in the case of a new pharmaceutical product, which is often designed to enter into and alter metabolic systems, than in the case of an industrial pollutant which simply happens to be passing through. Again, this is not a cast-iron distinction, with many pollutants having a much more dramatic toxic effect than the average pharmaceutical or food additive.

The fourth step involves so-called 'sub-acute' toxicity tests, in which repeated doses are typically given over a period of perhaps ninety days. In such tests, it is usual to start dosing the experimental animals shortly after they are weaned, with the dosing continuing through a period of rapid body growth. Both males and females are studied, with the animals allocated to treatment and control groups.

In addition to rats and mice, some researchers have used such species as dogs, hamsters, monkeys and rabbits in sub-acute toxicity studies. The problem with dogs and monkeys, as far as the researcher is concerned, is that they are expensive to breed and maintain, so that only relatively few animals can be used – and it can take longer than ninety days to cover their period of rapid growth properly. There are also more public protests about the experimental use of large mammals than there are about small mammals such as rats and mice.

Again, any effects of behaviour and health are noted, along with information on trends in body weight, consumption of food and water, the biochemistry of the animal's blood and urine, and the shape, structure and weight of its organs after its death.

The fifth step involves long-term toxicity studies, which will often focus on the development of tumours – itself a manifestation of chronic toxicity. 'Cancer,' as the chief medical officer at Britain's Department of Health and Social Security once put it, 'is one of the most emotive subjects with which the medical profession has to contend. Despite the significant advances that have been made in its treatment,' Dr Yellowlees warned, 'many problems remain over the detection of potential carcinogens.'

Carcinogens can affect us when taken through the mouth, inhaled, or absorbed through the skin. Tests for carcinogenicity are recommended where the chemical has a structure which suggests that it may be a carcinogen; where earlier studies of its action suggest that its pattern of toxicity or retention in the body is suspicious; or where large numbers of people are or may be exposed, or smaller groups are or may be heavily exposed.

One phenomenon of which researchers have become increasingly aware is 'co-carcinogenesis'. Agents which enhance the activity of carcinogens or magnify their effect can cause just as great a threat as those agents which actually trigger the cancer process. The problem is that many different types of process are often involved and appropriate test systems have yet to be developed, so that the regulatory authorities have so far tended to steer away from requiring detailed co-carcinogenesis studies. It is also worth pointing out that tumours found in test animals may not be caused by the chemical being tested, but may be triggered by the exposure of the animals to a virus or environmental mutagen during handling or administration of the chemical.

Because all species of animal spontaneously develop cancers, even when not exposed to the particular suspect chemical, tests for carcinogenicity have to be designed very carefully indeed. The animals in treatment and control groups are selected by a random procedure, but are similar in every respect, including age, sex, pre-natal and post-natal environment, body weight and so on. Once the experiment has actually begun, the animals have to be handled, caged and fed in exactly the same way, and any substance used to administer the chemical to them should itself be tested for toxic effects. In some cases, too, where the experiments involve an addition to the animal's diet, it is vitally important to know that all the animals are eating the same amount, as otherwise an effect associated with animals eating more or less than the average could be confused with the specific effect of an addition to their diet.

Once the study is completed, the researcher has to compare the observed number of different types of tumour in the animals exposed to the chemical with the number which might reasonably have been expected. If the number of tumours expected is sub-tracted from the number actually found, then we have a fairly crude indicator of carcinogenicity. However, statistical methods have evolved very rapidly and there are a growing number of tests for statistical significance. One of the most useful indicators is the test which matches increasing or decreasing dosage amounts or frequency with the trend in tumour formation. Although we shall be returning to the question of test accuracy, it is worth pointing out here that, if you are concerned about effects in people, the best test animal is the human. Most of the known human carcinogens have also been found to be carcinogenic in one experimental animal or another, but there is no evidence to prove that all animal carcinogens are also human carcinogens.

Whatever the problems encountered in animal tests, no battery of toxicity tests for a chemical likely to affect large numbers of people would now be complete without studies of its reproductive toxicity. The thalidomide tragedy and the various other repro-ductive problems and issues reviewed earlier have all helped ensure that reproductive toxicologists are included in the risk assessment team, particularly where women of childbearing age are likely to be exposed to the chemical.

Reproductive toxicologists typically divide their work into two main types: single-generation studies and multigeneration studies. The single-generation tests were devised as part of the response to the thalidomide tragedy, while the multigeneration tests have been largely developed to cover food additives and materials such as pesticides or residues from packaging which may become food contaminants.

A typical single-generation test programme might include two separate types of test. The first would involve the exposure of the male test animals for sixty days prior to mating, while the female animals were exposed for fourteen days. Later, the females would be exposed to the suspect chemical throughout their pregnancy. Half of the pregnant animals would be killed half-way through pregnancy, to see whether they had reabsorbed any embryos or whether any of the embryos they were carrying were abnormal in any way. The rest of the pregnant animals would be allowed to give birth, and their offspring would be killed and examined after they were weaned. This test reveals any effects on fertility and breeding performance. It may also help pinpoint any problems in foetal development, birth or lactation, unless the fact that the mother has been subjected to prolonged exposure has enabled her body to develop new routes for detoxifying the chemical.

In the second test, the key interests are embryotoxicity and teratogenicity, the pregnant animal being dosed with the chemical only during the period (between day 6 and day 15 for a rat) when the embryo is developing its organs. The pregnant animals are killed just before they are due to give birth, to check whether any of their embryos have been reabsorbed and their young are stained and sectioned with a razor, to check for any effects on their development. A third possible test would involve only dosing the pregnant animal late in pregnancy, to pinpoint any effects which are confined to the late stages of pregnancy or to the lactation period.

During these tests, it is vital that the pregnant animals be carefully treated, since such extraneous factors as noise or rough handling could significantly affect the outcome of the experiments. Reproductive toxicologists are also now advised to avoid an over-concentration on gross physical abnormalities, such as those produced by teratogens such as thalidomide. The field of embryo-toxicity, of which teratogenicity studies are one part, also includes the death of the foetus, any retardation of its growth and any upsets in its metabolism. Any researcher who focuses on gross abnormalities, it is increasingly felt, may be distracted from more subtle effects resulting from exposure to the suspect chemical.

Multigeneration studies are much less common than such

single-generation studies, but may be thought necessary where human exposure is likely to continue for some considerable period of time. They also permit the study of the behaviour of test animals exposed to the suspect chemical in the womb, a field of research which is becoming increasingly important.

Stripped to its bare essentials, this type of test involves the treatment or exposure of young male and female animals for about two months, after which they are mated and allowed to produce two litters. The offspring in the first litter are killed and examined after weaning, while the second litter form the parents of the next generation. These parents, in turn, are allowed to produce two litters, the second of which goes on to form the third generation of parents. Their two litters are also sacrificed on toxicology's altar. This process is carried out with three or more communities of animal, each of which is subjected to different levels of exposure.

This type of test is clearly going to be very expensive, and can take up to two years to complete. The EEC Sixth Amendment on dangerous substances requires such three-generation studies only for chemicals produced in quantities over 1,000 tonnes a year, or 5,000 tonnes in total, *if* some effect has been observed on fertility in smaller-scale tests run for lower levels of production. There has been considerable debate whether a two-generation study would not be equally acceptable: it would certainly be cheaper.

Overall, it can be said that such animal tests are fairly good at identifying the reproductive toxicity problems we now know about. On occasion, as with dibromochloropropane (DBCP), reproductive problems first emerged in test animals and the predictions about possible human effects made on the basis of these observations proved spot on. The US Environmental Protection Agency banned the use of DBCP in 1979, except in a number of Hawaiian pineapple plantations operated by Maui Pineapple Co. – but announced early in 1984 that it would ban this use as well, because of aquifer (groundwater) contamination.

The rodent studies on DBCP had highlighted a number of effects, including the atrophy of testicles and decreased fertility, with testicular atrophy, decreased sperm counts and decreased fertility also being found in people exposed to the chemical which was used as a soil fumigant and nematocide.

But experimental animals can react in very different ways from people. On the surface, it is obvious that their sexual behaviour is different from ours: sheep, for example, are seasonal breeders, while rabbits ovulate only after intercourse has taken place. But there may be deeper differences, too. Aspirin, for example, is often used in animal tests as a teratogen, or 'positive control teratogen', to use the jargon. One control group of animals is dosed with aspirin to see if they come up with the expected number of birth defects. But, despite a number of large epidemiological studies, no evidence of teratogenic effects has been found in humans.

The seventh major element in the toxicological detective work on a suspect chemical focuses on mutagenicity, or its ability to cause genetic mutations. The problem with mutations is that they can be transmitted from cell to cell during cell division or, even more worrying, from individual to individual via sexual reproduction.

When the Committee on Chemical Mutagens of the US National Research Council's Board on Toxicology and Environmental Health Hazards reviewed this field it found that there had been 'enormous progress in the development of simple, inexpensive, quick, sensitive and reproducible tests for mutagenicity. This progress,' it concluded, 'has resulted not only from the great interest in chemical mutagens since the 1960s, but also from the great increase in our fundamental understanding of genetics and molecular biology.'

The test system used most often is based on the bacterium *Salmonella*, with the Ames test, developed by Dr Bruce Ames and his co-workers, probably being the most popular. The basic idea in this type of test, which is designed to detect 'reverse mutations', is that the bacteria have mutations that prevent them from synthesizing histidine. Unless they have histidine, they cannot grow. Exposed to a mutagen, they may undergo a reverse mutation which enables them to start growing without histidine – and when they do so, the colony of mutated bacteria soon becomes obvious in what is otherwise a bacterial desert.

Two other types of bacterial test, based on the detection of forward mutations or of changes in bacterial DNA-damage repair systems, are less widely used. The strains of bacteria used are typically highly susceptible to the particular type of mutation which is being investigated. Because it is now recognized that many innocuous substances may become mutagenic only if activated by enzymes in the body, many bacterial tests now also include such enzymes, to activate the mutagens. Such tests can be completed within a few days, which obviously accounts for a good deal of their popularity.

Also increasingly popular are a number of mammalian cell strains which have been developed in such a way that they strongly encourage the growth of any mutant cells. One such system uses mouse lymphoma cells and is able to detect mutations causing a deficiency of thymidine kinase, while another uses Chinese hamster cells and detects mutations in the gene that produces HGPRT – which is shorthand for hypoxanthine-guanine phosphoribosyl transferase. They take longer than bacterial tests, generally being completed in a few weeks, but they offer a number of advantages and can also be used to test for chromosomal mutations.

Tests in the fruit-fly *Drosophila* also take a few weeks, but they afford a major advantage: an enormous amount is known about the genetics of this fly, which has been used to detect mutagens for more than fifty years. It is also a sexually reproducing eukaryotic organism which has male and female germ cells similar to those found in mammals. It also has a generation time of twelve days and each pair of parents can produce hundreds of offspring.

The test animal which is perhaps most useful is the mouse. Tests such as the 'specific-locus' test, the 'dominant-skeletal-mutation' test, or the 'cataract mutation' test have already produced a great deal of useful information on potential human mutagens. Another widely used mouse test is the 'dominant-lethal' test, which sets out to quantify embryo deaths in the womb which are caused by chromosomal damage. It is cheap and easy, but there is a high rate of spontaneous embryonic death in mice.

The American study concluded that 'the greatest difficulty with test systems today is that the tests that are most economical and sensitive use cell cultures or, if they use whole animals, use animals that are phylogenetically distant from man. In contrast, tests that use the mouse in ways that are directly comparable with the presumed human experience are too expensive to use for more than a small number of chemicals.'

To ensure accuracy in mutagen identification at reasonable cost, a two-tier test system was proposed for the USA. In the first tier, three tests would be used: a bacterial system and two mammalian cell systems, one designed to identify gene mutations and the other to identify chromosome breakages. If all three of these tests prove negative, the previously suspect chemical would be classified as a non-mutagen. If any two prove positive, the chemical would be classified as a mutagen, whereas if only one proved positive the second tier of testing would come into play, focusing on *Drosophila*. But both in the USA and in Europe, it has been felt that a test *in vivo*, in a live mammal, is also necessary if the chemical in question is in wide use, or is likely to be so.

The whole area of research on mutagens was given a major boost when new research supported an idea which had been out of fashion for some time, the idea that many cancers could have a genetic origin. Chromosomal abnormalities had been observed in tumours as early as 1914, but the idea that mutations could cause cancer was badly hit during the 1950s when known carcinogens, among them the polycyclic hydrocarbons, aromatic amines and azo-dyes, failed to induce mutations in the bacterial and other tests then used. The discovery that if some chemical carcinogen was mixed in with both bacteria and a preparation of liver enzymes they acted as bacterial mutagens indicates that the human metabolism itself was an important factor – and a factor which had generally been omitted from the earlier tests. In the mid-1970s, Ames and his colleagues reported the assay of 300 chemicals for mutagenicity in bacteria, using the new approach, and a 90 per cent correlation between carcinogenesis and mutagenesis was claimed.

Some known carcinogens, like asbestos and some hormones, are not thought to be mutagens, but there has been growing interest in the other side of the coin: how many of the 3,000 known mutagens are also carcinogens? One chemical which is being studied with particular interest is the food additive AF2, or trans-2-(2-furyl)-3-(nitro-2-furyl) acrylamide, widely used in Japan between 1964 and 1973 but abruptly withdrawn once it was shown to be a mutagen in animal tests. Later, longer-term studies also showed it to be an animal carcinogen, but it is too early as yet to tell whether it will prove to be a human carcinogen too.

The apparently strong links between mutagenicity and carcinogenicity have ensured that mutagenicity research has been underwritten to a much greater extent than it might have been had the only fear been that some chemicals might produce mutations. But all these animal, bacterial and other test systems suffer from a number of basic problems, including their use of organisms other than the one we are really interested in, and the fact that they often produce results based on the exposure of unusually sensitive organisms to unusually high doses of the suspect chemical.

The use of hyper-sensitive animals is justified on the basis that only a relatively small number of test animals can be used. A great deal of valuable work is going on into alternative, non-animal test methods, but the alternatives available are not really a substitute for animal tests. Instead they offer an early form of screening, to pick suspects for screening in animals. Even animal tests, however, are a second-best option, but an option which is forced upon us because there are very good ethical reasons for not using people, especially where the interest is in irreversible cancers or mutations.

The cost of the various tests can be very high. When Britain's Royal Society produced a report on risk assessment in 1983, it concluded that to test a food additive for acute toxicity, subchronic toxicity, chronic (i.e. lifetime) effects to establish no-effect levels (expressed in milligrams per kilogram), metabolic fate, carcinogenicity, reproductive toxicity and genetic toxicity would cost about £500,000. It also pointed out that 'if salt and sugar were considered to be potential (but unused) food additives, and were to be the subject of this spectrum of laboratory experiments in animals, and judgements were to be based purely upon the toxicological results, it is unlikely that either substance would be permitted for use in food!'

Ultimately, directly or indirectly, consciously or unconsciously, any chemical cleared in such tests is going to be tested on people, out in the real world. The Royal Society used the salt and sugar examples to illustrate its conclusion that 'We do not seem to be able today to make more accurate estimates of "risk-to-man" than we were twenty-five years ago when modern toxicology began to develop.' Part of the problem is clearly that, at the exposures typically encountered, it may be decades before significant health effects appear in those people exposed, by which time those effects may be aggravated or obscured by other factors, including the ageing process. But the fundamental difficulties involved in extrapolating from animal tests to the likely effects in people are equally important.

Any information we can get on the actual effects of particular chemicals on real people in the real world is obviously going to be very welcome indeed. Among the options open to us are the sort of clinical trials increasingly used on healthy human volunteers during the testing of new drugs and the long-term research of epidemiologists on the patterns of ill-health in populations or groups of individuals exposed to particular chemicals. Some of the detective work involved is described in Chapter 9, but first we need to look rather more carefully at another aspect of the toxicity question. So far we have been looking at the chemicals and other agents which can cause ill-health, in an attempt to understand what sorts of effects they might have on our health and why. But we also need to understand why different people exposed to the same chemical in similar conditions can show radically different reactions.

After the Falklands war, a great deal of attention was focused on the precision with which Exocet missiles homed in on their targets, wreaking a surprising amount of damage on some of the ships they hit. In the same way, toxicologists have often tended to be mesmerized by the incoming chemical rather than thinking about why the target responds in the way it does. The naval experts who had to carry out the post-mortems on the sunken and damaged ships knew they had to ask a different set of questions at the same time. Why were the incoming missiles able to penetrate the surveillance and defensive screens? And why, once they had hit their targets, were they able to reduce some warships to fiercely blazing hulks in a surprisingly short space of time?

Toxicologists are now asking the same questions about carcinogens, mutagens and teratogens. Why is it, they ask, that some people's immune systems can be penetrated much more easily than those of their siblings, workmates or neighbours? And why, once they have penetrated these defences, do some chemicals have such dramatically different effects on different people? Some of the answers are beginning to emerge from genetic screening research, a subject we will consider in the next chapter.

CHAPTER EIGHT

GENE SCREENS

If you were a butcher and you were considering hiring someone to work at the sharp end of the business, would you employ a haemophiliac? Think very carefully before you answer: once you have decided to exclude one set of people from a potentially hazardous occupation because of anomalies in their genetic make-up, you may find it increasingly difficult to know where to draw the line. Genetic screening, which involves testing the potential human victims rather than suspect chemicals or other challenges, is a technique which will be the subject of growing publicity (and controversy) through the 1980s and 1990s. It will impose increasingly hard choices not only on employers and employees, but also on would-be parents and parents-to-be.

Let's start with the employment picture. In 1982, the US Office of Technology Assessment (OTA) sent questionnaires to the chief executives of the 500 largest industrial companies in America, and to the top fifty utilities and eleven major labour unions. The American Industrial Health Council, an association of some 120 companies and eighty trade associations, circulated its members with a letter describing the questionnaire as 'objectionable' – although William J. McCarville, director of environmental affairs for Monsanto, later said that the letter had not been designed to dissuade the Council's members from filling in the forms. Whatever the truth of the matter, the OTA managed to achieve a 65 per cent overall response rate.

The survey results caused an uproar. Eighteen companies reported having used genetic screening techniques on their employees, or on potential recruits, during the previous five years, and fifty-four said that they planned to begin some genetic screening within the following five years. These testers and potential testers included chemical companies, oil companies, and manufacturers of rubber, plastics, metals and electronic components.

The OTA had promised respondents total anonymity, but some of the companies already employing genetic screening were well known. E. I. du Pont de Nemours & Co. was one of these and its screening programme was, to say the least, open to misinterpretation. Some of its critics alleged that the company's screens for employees with genes predisposing them to sickle cell anaemia was simply a ruse to exclude blacks from employment in the chemical industry.

Du Pont, however, insisted that the facts of the case were less controversial. It had been approached in 1972 by its own Black Du Pont Employees Association to launch a screening programme for sickle cell genes among its black employees. But the company pointed out that the tests were entirely voluntary; that black employees could refuse to take the tests if they so wished, without affecting their employment prospects; and, more important, even those found to have genes predisposing them to sickle cell anaemia were not denied employment. 'Workers in whom we find these traits,' said the director of the company's Haskell Laboratory for Toxicology and Industrial Medicine, 'are offered placement in areas where they cannot come in contact with the hazardous chemicals.'

To understand why some employees might feel sensitive about such tests, it helps to know something about the history of those tests and about the circumstances in which they might be used. Two main types of genetic test have been used on employees of US chemical corporations to date: *genetic screening* and *genetic monitoring.* The purpose of genetic screening, in industry at least, is to pinpoint those people who have inherited a trait which may predispose them to illness when exposed to some environmental 'trigger', such as a workplace chemical. In genetic monitoring programmes, on the other hand, employees are checked for genetic damage after some exposure to such agents has taken place.

The screening test used by Du Pont measures levels of an enzyme found in human red blood cells, known as glucose-6-phosphate dehydrogenase (or G-6-PD). Men, and typically they are of African or Mediterranean descent, may inherit a deficiency of G-6-PD which may confer some protection against malaria but also, it turns out, prevents them from metabolizing some drugs and some of the chemicals used in manufacturing explosives and chemical dyes. When exposed to such chemicals, men who suffer from G-6-PD deficiency can develop severe anaemia, although the response to such exposure varies widely.

In genetic monitoring programmes, scientists look for breakages and other abnormalities in the chromosomes of industrial employees. But they run into real difficulties when it comes to interpreting the data they have collected. Sunbathing, medication and viral infections can all cause chromosome breakages, which means that the 'background' level of anomalies can show significant natural fluctuations. Teasing out the effects of a particular workplace chemical can be a highly fraught exercise, both because workers are rarely exposed to just one chemical and because science has yet to demonstrate any really conclusive link between such anomalies and health problems such as cancer.

One of the better known genetic monitoring programmes was that run (and later dropped) by Dow Chemical. In 1977, during a programme which ran for more than ten years, Dow monitored the chromosomes of employees working with benzene and epichlorohydrin, both of which were thought to be carcinogenic at high exposure levels. Benzene has not shown up as a mutagen in bacterial test systems, and tests on pregnant mice, rats and rabbits have shown no embryolethal or teratogenic effects even where the dose was sufficient to kill the pregnant animal itself. Women have proved more susceptible to benzene poisoning than men, perhaps because there is greater uptake and storage in fat. Benzene does cross the placenta, however, and may be present in foetal blood at levels equal to or even exceeding those in the mother's blood. Some investigators have found an increased abortion rate in exposed female workers, although there appears to have been little research into the effect of benzene exposure on male or female fertility. Chromosomal damage has been reported, although chromosomal changes were apparently not found at exposures below 15 parts per million.

Epichlorohydrin, which like benzene is used as an industrial solvent, has been shown to depress the fertility of male rats and it is unquestionably mutagenic both in bacterial test systems and in mammalian systems, including exposed workers. There have also been suggestions that there may be a respiratory carcinogenic effect in exposed workers, and the Guy's Hospital Medical School team drew attention to the urgent need for more human studies.

Given the industrial importance of these two chemicals, and the numbers of workers exposed throughout the chemical industry in particular, there was dismay at Dow when its research identified what seemed to be increased chromosomal breakages among employees known to have histories of relatively low exposure to the chemicals. 'The normal breakage rate varies so much,' Dow's medical director explained later, 'it was hard to see if there was a real problem.' The monitoring programme was dropped in the midst of a fairly acrimonious debate about the significance of the results reported.

Dow has since been investigating the normal fluctuations in background chromosome damage, and says that it may resume genetic monitoring if it can work out a way to make sense of its data. Meanwhile, a number of new tests are being developed, one of which measures the inherited activity level of an enzyme which detoxifies the pesticide parathion and perhaps also malathion, the pesticide used in California against Medfly infestations after the failure (through incompetence, rather than because of any intrinsic weakness in biological pest control systems) of a biological pest control programme. Apparently about half the population of the United States inherits a low-activity form of the relevant enzyme and half a high-activity form – a fact which ought to be of considerable interest to anyone handling such chemicals or employing others to do so.

Surprisingly, when the US National Institute of Occupational Health and Safety (NIOSH) completed a three-year study of the industries which were most likely to report high cancer rates among their workers, it found that the major chemical companies ranked low on the list, in twelfth place.

Top of the list came companies producing industrial and scientific instruments, presumably because workers in this industry work with such hazardous materials as asbestos, solder and thallium. Consider thallium. It is used for a fairly wide range of applications, from rodent poisons through semiconductor pro- duction to uses in switches and closures operating at sub-zero temperatures, typically as an alloy with mercury. Interestingly, although thallium is known to cross the placenta in rodents, cats and humans, the Guy's Hospital Medical School team found no reputable studies on carcinogenicity or mutagenicity. In fact it drew attention to the lack of data not only in respect of the possibility that thallium could act either as a carcinogen or a mutagen, but also in respect of its reproductive toxicology.

After instrument manufacturers, NIOSH reported, came a cluster of companies using such materials as asbestos, chromic acid, lead, nickel and solvents to manufacture metal products. Other industries which had the unhappy distinction of appearing in the NIOSH top ten were those producing electrical equipment (which can involve exposure to lead, mercury, solder and solvents); leather products (involving exposure to chrome salts and other tanning chemicals); machinery (cutting and lubricating oils); equipment used in the transport industry (where plastics are often used, including such constituents as formaldehyde); and those building pipelines (oil derivatives and welding materials).

Critics of the study pointed out that NIOSH has only looked for chemicals which were known to cause cancer, or strongly suspected of doing so. Industries which use chemicals which may yet emerge as potent carcinogens obviously were not included, nor were those using materials already known to cause serious health problems other than cancer.

One thing can be almost guaranteed, however, and that is that any company announcing that it intends to improve its health and safety performance by developing a genetic screening programme will find itself under intense scrutiny by those who would prefer to see it clean up the industrial environment instead. Yet, as Dr Thomas Murray of the Hastings Center, Hastings-on-Hudson, New York, has said the basic idea underlying genetic screening 'seems remarkably simple and humane. Not everyone exposed to a health hazard gets sick, so why not protect people who are especially susceptible to the hazard by keeping them away from it?' Or, as *Chemical Week* put it in an editorial, 'It makes no economic sense to spend millions of dollars to tighten up a process that is dangerous only for a tiny fraction of employees – if the susceptible individuals can be identified and isolated from it.'

Murray traced the idea back at least as far as 1938, when J. B. S. Haldane, the English geneticist who first established the rate of mutation of a human gene, wrote that 'the majority of potters do not die of bronchitis. It is quite possible that if we really understood the causation of this disease we should find that only a fraction of potters are of a constitution which renders them liable to it. If so, we could eliminate potters' bronchitis by regulating entrants into the potters' industry who are congenitally predisposed to it.'

Two more recent proponents of genetic screening, Dr Zsolt Harsanyi and Richard Hutton, traced the idea even further back, to the observation by Sir Percival Potts that only some chimney sweeps in eighteenth-century England contracted scrotal cancer as a result of their occupation. As they pointed out, the automatic reaction of anyone diagnosed to have a disease which appears to strike more or less at random is: 'Why me?' Genetic screening is already providing some answers.

One striking conundrum was resolved by a genetic screening programme in Sardinia during the 1950s, a success which inspired many later efforts. Up to 35 per cent of the island's population at that time suffered from mysterious symptoms. The reported symptoms ranged from lethargy to death. The problem turned out to be haemolytic anaemia and the culprit was identified as that same defective G-6-PD gene, a gene which had become widespread in Sardinia's relatively pure human gene pool. It emerged that only those who carried the defective gene and who then ate raw or partly cooked fava beans (or breathed the pollen from fava plants) came down with the disease.

Two years after this discovery was made, a simple blood test was developed at the University of Washington which could measure the presence or absence of G-6-PD. 'Armed with the test,' Harsanyi and Sutton recall, 'scientists now had a way of determining exactly who was predisposed to the disease and who was not. The missing enzyme had become a tool of prediction, a signal that the disease might someday strike.'

G-6-PD, then, was an early example of what is now known as a 'genetic marker', enabling doctors to identify people likely to develop haemolytic anaemia when exposed to such triggers as fava bean pollen, anti-malarial drugs, aspirin or even vitamin K.

The problem is that any given genetic marker may take years, even decades, to identify. A group of chemicals which illustrates this fact is the arylamines, which are still used in the manufacture of hair dyes, pigments, plastics, rubber and textiles. The first person to suspect that arylamines could be carcinogenic was the German physician Ludwig Rehn, who spotted the fact that workers in the synthetic dye industry were showing much higher rates of bladder cancer than other industrial workers, let alone the population as

a whole. This was in 1895. It took four decades before scientists
were able to show that arylamine caused bladder cancer in dogs
– and a further fifteen years before research in the British dye
industry came up with conclusive proof that arylamines cause
human cancers.

Even this was not the end of the story. As Harsanyi and Sutton
pointed out, 'implicating arylamines did little good. Not every dye
worker develops cancer, even under similar working conditions.
At first, researchers believed that the differences might be due to
dietary habits. But soon other pieces of the puzzle began to fall into
place. Animal experiments clearly showed that arylamines were
not dangerous in themselves; they had to be transformed by the
body into carcinogens.'

Humans can transform arylamines, so risking cancer. Dogs,
which were used in many of the tests, are even more at risk; yet
guinea pigs, which are frequently used in such tests, cannot transform arylamine – and therefore are much less at risk. As research
continued, however, it became clear that there are considerable
variations in the reaction of different groups of people to arylamine
exposure. These variations, it emerged, reflect the extent to which
different people can produce an enzyme called N-acetyltransferase
(NAT). NAT, it was discovered, targets arylamines, straps a
further chemical to them and, in doing so, defuses these potent
carcinogens.

If you are the sort of person who can produce NAT in the
necessary amounts, you would be described as a 'rapid acetylator'.
If not, consider yourself a slow acetylator – and steer clear of arylamines. Anyone who is a slow acetylator, with low NAT levels, is
clearly at a greater risk of contracting cancer. When scientists
began to screen large numbers of people for NAT activity, they
came up with some interesting results. The Caucasian population
of North America, for example, was found to be almost exactly split
between slow and rapid acetylators. It was also found that whereas
50 per cent of North American Caucasians were slow acetylators,
the numbers ran as low as 10 per cent among Orientals and as high
as 70 per cent among Israelis.

The question now is whether NAT activity can be more widely
used as a genetic marker? One scientist who has argued that it
could be is G. M. Lower of the University of Wisconsin. When he
visited Denmark, where the ratio of slow to rapid acetylators is

about the same as that found in the United States, he tested cancer patients drawn from the urban population of Copenhagen. His results were striking: twice as many slow acetylators turned up among those he studied, suggesting that slow acetylators, if they are city-dwellers, may be twice as likely to contract cancer. Lower was not immediately able to track down the cause of this imbalance, but his working hypothesis was that arylamines must be much more widespread in the typical urban environment than they are in country areas – a conclusion which was supported by the absence of any marked difference between slow and rapid acetylators living and working in rural areas.

The techniques which underpin genetic screening programmes are evolving rapidly, although it is interesting to note that as late as 1982, in testimony before the Subcommittee on Investigations and Oversight of the US House of Representatives, Dr Thomas Murray argued that 'despite the enthusiasm of early proponents, scientific experts today agree nearly unanimously that there are *no* solid candidates for screening today'.

Murray recalled the influential paper written in the early 1960s by H. E. Stokinger and L. D. Scheel which had the following to say about the implications of the G-6-PD test: 'Most important, the determination affords, for the first time, an opportunity to make a susceptibility evaluation during the job placement examination and, thus, avoids placing a worker in exposures to which he is inordinately susceptible. This is preventative toxicology in the highest form; no previous single development in toxicology has opened such prospects for the medical supervision of workers.'

Ten years later, in 1973, Herbert Stokinger joined forces with another co-author, John Mountain, to publish what was, as Dr Murray suggests, 'misleadingly titled a "consensus report"'. This listed five candidates for 'hypersusceptibility' screens: G-6-PD, sickle cell trait, alpha-1-antitrypsin deficiency (possibly predisposing those with the deficiency to emphysema, a chronic lung condition), and two conditions with less defined genetic bases: reactions to carbon disulphide and to organic cyanates such as toluene diisocyanate.

And then, nearly ten years later again, a revised list was published by Gilbert Omenn which recommended that G-6-PD, alpha-1-antitrypsin deficiency and immune reactions to isocyanates be subjected to further study, together with a few additional conditions. Omenn cautioned, 'No genetic screening tests should be applied routinely at this time.' But, as Murray hurried to point out, 'genetic screening is going on already and it will continue to be done, whether or not the experts believe it is scientifically valid. Even those who say the science is not ripe admit that this is merely a temporary condition, soon to be remedied.'

Harsanyi and Hutton were even more confident that genetic screening would soon be available almost over the counter. Medical science, they suggested, 'is now on the verge of developing a comprehensive system of predicting and preventing diseases by analysing each individual's own particular set of genetic markers'. Within ten years, they believed, 'anybody will be able to go into a local clinic, have a blood sample taken and receive a computer print-out of their susceptibilities to scores of diseases'.

New techniques such as trophoblast sampling are already enabling some parents in high-risk groups to check foetuses for a growing number of serious congenital conditions – even for damage perhaps caused by mutagens. Previously, the sampling of the amniotic fluid surrounding the foetus in the womb could only be attempted after eighteen weeks of a pregnancy, by which point, as one of the developers of trophoblast sampling put it, 'a child feels far more like a little human than it does at eight weeks'.

Some communities, such as Britain's Cypriot community, have embraced genetic screening, together with late abortions of affected foetuses for particularly serious ailments. In this case the main problem is thalassaemia, which requires nightly medication and monthly blood transfusions. The Asian community, affected by the same problem, have rejected abortions, although some now believe that these latest techniques, which permit sampling when the foetus is only nine weeks old, will circumvent some of the religious principles involved. At this point, the foetus is less than two centimetres long, which previously made sampling impossible without damaging the foetus itself. But the trophoblast, the webby filaments which surround the foetus and later develop into the placenta, *can* be sampled – and proves to have the same genetic composition as the foetus.

Inevitably such successes, while they may come as a boon to parents who would otherwise have to raise a child with an incurable condition, have stirred fierce controversy. 'I can see no difference between seeking out mongol children in the womb to kill them and putting them into gas chambers after birth,' said Professor John Scarisbrick, chairman of the British anti-abortion organization, Life. 'Either they are human beings or they are not.'

Ultimately, gene therapy may be possible, involving the remoulding of some aspects of an embryo's genetic make-up before it is even born. The idea underlying what has been called 'genetic surgery' has been that recombinant DNA techniques would be used to snip out 'bad' genes and insert 'good' ones in their place. Late in 1982, however, the *New England Journal of Medicine* carried a report which suggested that another route might be practicable.

A new method, developed by scientists at the National Heart, Lung and Blood Institute in Bethesda, Maryland, the University College of Illinois College of Medicine in Chicago and Johns Hopkins University in Baltimore, had used a drug to reactivate genes which had apparently been dormant since birth. Originally tested in baboons, the method had been used on a handful of patients suffering from severe thalassaemia or sickle cell anaemia. Both these blood disorders result from defects in the genes which control the production of haemoglobin. Thalassaemia victims cannot produce healthy red blood cells, which is why they need regular blood transfusions. Those with sickle cell anaemia, on the other hand, experience painful blood vessel blockages.

The drug used was 5-azacytidine, which had previously been used in cancer therapy. One thalassaemia patient, who had needed a transfusion every two weeks, received a continuous infusion of the drug for seven days. By the seventh day, his blood contained 25 per cent more healthy red blood cells than it did before therapy began. This effect lasted for about a month. The scientists involved in the research were not at all sure how the therapy was actually achieving its beneficial effect, although they speculated that the drug was stripping the relevant genes of some chemical which had suppressed their activity, switching them on again. The genes in question produce haemoglobin in the foetus and are replaced by a second set of genes after birth, although it is not clear why this transfer takes place.

Such techniques will inevitably bring their own risks. One patient who underwent this form of therapy, for example, reported feeling transient nausea and vomiting. Despite claims that the technique demonstrated 'beyond doubt', as haematologist Dr Edward Benz of Yale University School of Medicine put it in an editorial accompanying the original announcement of the research results, that 'genetic manipulation has come to the bedside', there were anxieties about the possible long-term effects of the therapy itself. Apart from the question of nausea and vomiting, there was an even more worrying issue: were other genes being altered by the 5-azacytidine, including possibly genes which predispose some people to cancer?

Genetic surgery and therapy will prove even more contentious than genetic screening. But, while genetic surgery and the various associated techniques will provide plenty of fodder for those whose business it is to consider the ethical implications of new medical breakthroughs, the rapid development of genetic screening technology will continue to tax those who have to make what could prove to be life-or-death decisions, whether they be parents or, as employers, guardians of their employees' health.

Apart from any emotional or ethical considerations, however, such techniques promise to be highly cost-effective, and they will therefore be adopted by many health authorities or industrial employers when they can be shown to be effective. The problem, and it was underscored by Dr Murray in his testimony, is that current test methods by no means guarantee accurate results. If you were faced with a condition found in one birth in a thousand, or in one worker in a thousand, and you developed a test which was 99 per cent accurate and no mistakes were made in applying the method, then you could hope to identify all ten true cases (or 'true positives') in a population of 10,000. But you would also identify a hundred 'false positives', people who could be denied employment (or foetuses which might be aborted) for no good reason.

Dr Murray suggested that the evidence about the linkages between a particular environmental challenge and a disease or impairment can be expected to appear in three distinct stages. First, clinical work on individual workers reveals a suspected connection between a genetic condition and an occupationally induced condition. These relatively vague and inconclusive suspicions will be followed by epidemiological studies of populations of workers exposed to the challenge, and of control groups who are not. Third, if these confirm the initial suspicions, pilot studies of screening techniques should follow, with initial screening followed by genetic monitoring, to see whether the predictions are borne out in practice.

According to Dr Murray, we have stage one evidence in a mere handful of cases, but there is as yet no really conclusive evidence for either stages two or three. More worryingly, there is evidence that some exclusionary policies already used by US employers have been ineffective. The lower back X-rays used in the railroad industry, for example, clear a population of workers who suffer the same rate of back injuries as those caught by the screen – and who are denied certain forms of employment as a direct result.

Once reliable data are in, however, employers have at least three options. They can choose to ignore the evidence and, if they are responsible, clean up the working environment instead. They can brief their workers on the risks and leave the decision to the individuals concerned. Or they can simply decide to exclude suspected high-risk people. Clearly these three options are by no means mutually exclusive, but if they take the third option in isolation, they may well find their exclusions running along racial and ethnic lines, reinforcing the obstacles facing those who already suffer from job discrimination.

Yet, as Dr Murray himself asked: 'Should we refuse to act paternalistically to protect a worker who appears to be making a deadly choice?' Much will depend, of course, on the actual risk run and on the severity of the potential outcome. Meanwhile, we will continue to uncover new and problematic links between genetics and environmental agents – links which even the affected employees may be inclined to ignore when acceptable alternative jobs are scarce or unavailable.

'The discovery of better and more accurate markers foreshadows the speedy expansion of industrial screening,' Harsanyi and Hutton concluded. But soon, they warned, 'we may find ourselves caught in an ever-tightening spiral: finding markers for more subtle problems, discovering larger numbers of susceptible workers, labelling more and different types of environment as hazardous. It is not inconceivable that, through screening, industry will become the modern counterpart of Diogenes, as it searches for the perfect worker.'

Interestingly, research has shown that 90 per cent of all workers participate in voluntary screening programmes in factories where they have been mounted, compared with perhaps 30 per cent in community programmes. And those who have considered the ethical implications of these new techniques, like researchers at the Hastings Center, have tended to conclude that the use of genetic tests to diagnose specific illnesses (or a predisposition to such illnesses) in individual workers is acceptable, but in making the case for their acceptability, Dr Murray insisted that a number of important pre-conditions should be met.

An absolute requirement, he suggested, is that there must be sound scientific evidence linking a particular genetic anomaly to demonstrated risk. Furthermore, he proposed, the relative and absolute risks involved (or suspected from the evidence in hand) should be very large. Misclassifications, resulting in false positives or negatives, should be few and reversible. The number of persons likely to be excluded should be very small. Very few jobs should be involved. The disease should be 'severe, irreversible and not readily diagnosed in its pre-clinical phases' and the programme 'should not single out already beleaguered groups'.

Even if all these pre-conditions are met, it should be recognized that genetic screening can help only where there is an undisputed genetic marker and where the potentially vulnerable group is a fairly small proportion of the population being considered. Many hazardous chemicals may affect different people at somewhat different rates and perhaps even in slightly different ways, but the fact remains that they are intrinsically harmful. Either no one should be exposed to them or, where exposure is inescapable, it should be kept to the absolute minimum – and certainly below the relevant safety standards. And the fact remains that some important diseases may yet prove to be caused by exposure to a number of chemicals, some of which sensitize those exposed to later chemicals, rather than to a single carcinogen, mutagen or teratogen. Step beyond the factory fence, into the real world of multiple exposures to an enormous variety of chemicals, most of them totally safe if considered in isolation, and the picture inevitably becomes even trickier.

Genetic screening, in short, is a partial answer to what, in the light of the evidence presented in previous chapters, must be considered the wrong question. If we ask how we can pinpoint those people with a hypersusceptibility to a single chemical, or a single family of chemicals, then genetic screening may well be able to provide answers. But if, on the other hand, we ask how we can ensure that the increasing exposure of increasing numbers of people to increasing numbers of chemicals does not result in belated identification of unsuspected carcinogens, mutagens or teratogens, then genetic screening can only be a relatively small part of the answer even if it achieves the targets that are being set for it. Other, and generally complementary, elements of a strategy for living in the alien environment we have created (and will continue to create) for ourselves are next on the agenda.

CHAPTER NINE

THE
TOXIC
FRONTIER

The chemical industry has a word for it. Chemophobia. The fear of chemicals has swept through country after country, community after community. The media, ready to publicize any adverse effects, has aroused the fears of communities which have concluded that they are a potential Seveso or the next Love Canal. Like the medieval witchcraft purges, these fears have fed upon themselves, with each successive toxic spill, plant explosion or unexplained rise in local cancer rates igniting more psychological fuses and increasing the pressure on politicians, on the regulatory agencies and on industry.

This unhappy state of affairs represents a complete reversal for the chemical industry. 'If there was one industry that perhaps best epitomized progress,' as the president of the Ciba-Geigy Corporation has put it, 'it was the chemical industry. Plastics, synthetic fibers, miracle drugs, elimination of pests, better crop production, the decline in disease, all these resulted in a cleaner, healthier, more comfortable, more convenient life. In short, I think we believed the well-known advertising slogan, "Better Living Through Chemistry". So what happened,' he asked, 'to change the positive into the negative? What made us aware of the price-tag associated with progress?'

Rachel Carson, in a word. Her book *Silent Spring* fuelled the explosive growth of the environmental movement, as she had always hoped it would. But the chemophobia of the 1960s and

1970s was also fuelled by a wider loss of confidence in industry in the wake of the Vietnam débâcle, the energy crisis, the rise of inflation, and of the successful campaigns launched by the environmental and consumer movements. The problems and phobias have often seemed worse in the United States than elsewhere, so it came as no surprise to hear William Ruckelshaus, shortly after he took over from the disgraced Anne Burford at the US Environmental Protection Agency, lament that the country was caught up in a feverish quest for the 'chemical of the month', with the limelight moving from DDT through PCBs to dioxin and new concerns such as ethylene dibromide – a pesticide and anti-knock compound used as a petrol additive, known to cause withering of the testicles in test animals.

Ciba-Geigy, in fact, had been one of the companies which had been calling for a much more sympathetic handling of chemicals and of the chemical industry by the media. 'Chemophobia has had a significant impact,' its president said, in a masterpiece of understatement. 'In the news media, with one-sided, negative stories. In the public's poor perception of the industry. In more burdensome regulation. In high costs and reduced productivity. In shorter patent life and lower returns on investments. In less research being done, and, ultimately, in fewer new drugs and other chemical products being introduced.'

All true, of course, and it is difficult not to sympathize with the view that 'it's time for the pendulum to swing back so that the benefits of chemicals as well as the risks are discussed, so that a more balanced story can be told and believed'. Even Rachel Carson took great pains to point out that she was not against the use of crop protection chemicals, but against their abuse. The spread of chemophobia is causing needless stress, as in the case of the phantom toxic leak in Memphis. 'There were all the usual details – reports of unusual diseases, picketing, emotional meetings, even a congressional hearing,' Jeremy Main recalls. 'The only thing lacking was a dump or other source of poisonous chemicals. It was never found and a study by the federal Centers for Disease Control determined eventually that there was no unusual incidence of illness.'

On the other hand, our increasingly sensitive environmental monitoring systems *are* picking up an increasing number of chemicals broadly dispersed in the environment. The scale of pollution in some regions of the world is phenomenal. Some 430 billion tonnes of domestic wastes are discharged into the Mediterranean each year, for example, with coastal industries contributing an estimated 5,000 tonnes of zinc, 1,400 tonnes of lead, 950 tonnes of chromium and 10 tonnes of mercury each year. In addition, the various rivers which flow into the Mediterranean add a further 100 tonnes of mercury, with the atmosphere now believed to dump perhaps four times as much mercury into this enclosed sea as do the rivers. And it is also estimated that some 90 tonnes of persistent pesticides find their way into the Mediterranean each year, along with some 800,000 tonnes of oil. Sadly, the Mediterranean is not an isolated example.

Opinions vary enormously as to the significance of the resulting human exposures to particular pollutants. Take the case of cadmium in Britain's soils and food, with the Ministry of Agriculture, Fisheries and Food being challenged by independent experts in its conclusion that dietary intakes are well below the 'tolerable' safety standards set by the World Health Organization (WHO). The Ministry reported that average weekly intakes of cadmium through food hover around the 140 milligrams mark, which is indeed well below the 400 milligrams WHO standard. But scientists at the Institute of Terrestrial Ecology, the London School of Economics, and St Thomas' Hospital, London, warned that this standard is probably unhealthily high and that those living or working in cadmium 'hot spots' are likely to be exposed to even higher levels of cadmium.

They found that only 40 parts per million of cadmium in animal kidney tissue could cause damage, a level which is less than a sixth of that considered safe by WHO. 'Cadmium is a cumulative poison, as is radiation,' said Dr Jeremy Nicholson of the London School of Economics. 'The more you have of it, the greater are the chances that something nasty will happen.' The resulting damage is not confined to the liver and kidneys, however, as Dr Marion Kendall of the anatomy department at St Thomas' Hospital has pointed out. 'The trouble with cadmium,' she said, 'is that it interferes with the body's control of zinc, and zinc is vital to cell functioning. Without it, normal cell manufacture and repair is seriously affected.' But would the results of the animal tests be paralleled in people? 'I will be very surprised,' she replied, 'if these findings are not confirmed in men and women.'

Industry has already spent a great deal of money on cutting its heavy metal discharges. Indeed, some companies are far from convinced that the money they have been forced to spend has been money well spent. In the wake of the Minamata disaster, for example, chemical companies around the world came under intense pressure to cut their mercury discharges. 'Undoubtedly we took the action we did willingly and it was considered right at the time,' said ICI's group environment adviser, Mike Flux. By 1982, ICI had spent some £25 million on capital projects designed to cut mercury discharges from the company's chlor-alkali plants, and had also incurred running costs estimated at £1.9 million. In addition, an extensive programme of environmental monitoring had been carried out by the company's Brixham Laboratory, which had cost something like £1 million over fifteen years. The conviction was growing in ICI that the money could have been better spent.

Over the period in question, it is certainly possible to show that the concentrations of mercury in fish in the Irish Sea fell from about 0.5 milligrams per kilogram (mg/kg) to under 0.3 mg/kg. Ever since the Minamata poisonings, the regulatory authorities have been particularly concerned about mercury levels in fish. 'All forms of mercury can be harmful once they have entered the body tissues,' said Flux. 'However, metallic and inorganic forms of mercury are only slowly absorbed and are relatively rapidly excreted. By contrast, organo-mercury compounds, and especially methyl mercury compounds, are readily absorbed and only slowly eliminated.' But why are we so worried about fish? The reason is that research studies have shown that some 90 per cent of the mercury found in fish occurs in its methyl form.

So what represents a safe level of mercury in fish? The fisheries industry would be hard pressed to tell you. The Americans and Canadians have decided that the limit should be 0.5 mg/kg, although after challenges in court from the tuna industry the practical limit in the United States was set at 1.0 mg/kg – and the industry kept pressing for 2.0 mg/kg. In the Mediterranean, the limit for tuna was set at 0.7 mg/kg.

In Japan, where the problem first hit the headlines, the regulators have taken into account the importance of fish in the diet of most Japanese and their low average body weight, and have come up with an even lower figure: 0.4 mg/kg. 'The EEC, not to be outdone,' Flux noted, 'and without explaining its rationale, decided on 0.3 mg/kg – apparently because the UK Government volunteered this figure, on the basis that it was aleady being achieved.'

A study carried out by the UK government, comparing a high-risk community with a fish consumption about seventeen times the national average – and that fish caught in mercury-contaminated waters – with a similar population eating fish taken from uncontaminated waters, showed that 13 per cent of the high-risk group had a mercury risk exceeding the WHO recommended level – even though the average mercury level, at 0.27 mg/kg, was just under the EEC limit. Interestingly, the 'worst case' individual, who consumed something like twice the recommended levels, had a blood mercury level which was still an order of magnitude lower than the level at which WHO expected to see symptoms in even the most sensitive members of the population.

'Even allowing for the uncertainties about possible effects on unborn children,' Flux concluded, 'this evidence suggests a very handsome margin of safety even for the highest risk members of any European community. There is also doubt about whether there would have been any significant risk even at the level obtaining before all this expensive activity took place.' There is, he suggested, a widespread feeling in the industry that 'a great deal of money has been spent to reduce mercury emission from the chlor-alkali industry without a commensurate benefit in the well-being of mankind, and that any residual real risk could have been contained for a much smaller sum. It is fascinating to speculate,' he said, 'what much clearer benefits might have been achieved by alternative uses of the large sums involved.' But, as he himself later pointed out, 'people don't want to spend money on "maybe" issues. They are only really happy to do so when an issue turns up on the doorstep.' The mercury issue turned up on the doorstep at ICI's Mond Division: it is difficult to see what else Mond could have done in the circumstances.

At least countries such as Britain have a fairly good idea of where the wastes they generate are going, which is more than can be said of rapidly industrializing countries such as Ireland. Because Ireland is a member of the EEC, it is being pressed into line, but the country's rapid industrial growth has raced well ahead of its ability to comprehend and control the pollution generated in the process. It is estimated, for example, that a total of 20,000 tonnes of toxic waste are generated in Ireland each year, with fully 5,000 tonnes of this waste 'disappearing', in the sense that they cannot be accounted for. The government's Institute for Industrial Research and Standards (IIRS) has been trying to track down the missing wastes.

No one doubts that industry throughout the developed world has made major strides in cleaning up its environmental performance in recent years; indeed most of us forget how low environmental protection came on any industrial list of priorities even as recently as the early 1970s. An extraordinary illustration of this is offered by Charles Brookes, senior vice-president for environmental policy at W. R. Grace & Co. One day, well over a decade ago, he was brought a set of aerial photographs of the company's Curtis Bay plant in Maryland, intended for office decoration. To his horror, he recalls, he and his staff found a 'two-square-mile red blotch staring at us', produced by a chemical Grace had been dumping into Chesapeake Bay. When Mr Brookes ordered a subordinate to 'do something about the pollution', the man repaired to his own office and returned later with a new set of photographs, with the red areas neatly airbrushed out. 'That was his solution,' Mr Brookes explains, adding that the employee in question later left the company. 'That was 1970,' he says. 'We didn't think about these things.'

As Bayer's achievements (described on pp. 157–9) show, a great deal can be done to cut the risks associated with toxic waste disposal. But, as Philip Palmer, a senior environmental engineer at Du Pont, has put it, any attempt to reduce the output of such wastes and ensure their safe disposal involves addressing 'a lot of different little problems'. The public, he says, harbour the illusion that it is possible to 'do something magic' about such wastes. In the real world, he stresses, there 'isn't going to be any single technical panacea'. Even so, the chemical industry now recognizes that the toxic waste disposal issue merits top priority, whether or not it gets it in particular companies. It has become, in the words of the Chemical Manufacturers Association, 'a motherhood issue'.

Motherhood issues, in fact, have been at the heart of an increasing number of major pollution controversies, including those which have taken California's Silicon Valley by storm. 'I can't say for sure it's their fault. I can't prove it yet,' said Mrs Mary Lou Lujan, who worked for Fairchild Camera and Instrument making microchips. 'But in myself I know my baby died because I was exposed to those chemicals and because I drank that water.' The chemicals she was talking about were those used in microchip production, some of which are extremely toxic. By 1979, Silicon Valley was using an astounding 64,000 cubic feet of arsine, the toxic gas used as a weapon in the First World War. Mrs Lujan's early symptoms had included headaches, drowsiness, and a constant thirst, which she slaked at Fairchild's drinking fountain. In the early months of her pregnancy she noticed 'horrible spots around my mouth; my mouth went very cold'. Her baby was born on 15 June 1981 with a perforated stomach and died five days later.

Six months later, Fairchild discovered that a storage tank under its plant had been leaking, contaminating a local well with 1,1,1-trichloroethane, a degreasing agent, used in the microchip industry, which can damage the central nervous system, liver and heart. The well served 16,500 households and 266 residents later sued Fairchild, alleging that the resulting pollution had caused miscarriages and heart defects among their children. 'The industry that can mount an electronic brain on a pinhead,' the press exclaimed, 'cannot stop its tanks from leaking.' Fairchild promptly spent $14 million trying to clean up, but test wells remained contaminated. A leak-proof tank and leak detection equipment would have cost $100,000.

The environmental authorities were stung into demanding that other Silicon Valley companies check for similar leaks. By mid-1983, sixty-seven companies had found contamination and further reports of leaks were coming in at the rate of one a week. Among the solvents involved were trichloroethylene, 1,1-dichloroethylene and perchloroethylene. Intel was one of the companies which reported a large leak of trichloroethylene (TCE or 'trike'), a highly toxic chemical which can readily cross the human placenta and is a suspected mutagen.

Among the 266 people initially suing Fairchild, there were twenty-two women who had suffered miscarriages, seven whose babies had died from congenital defects and eighteen whose children suffered from heart ailments. All this was a shocking reversal for the gleaming, high-technology industry, long considered 'squeaky clean'. State pollution officials had thought of the industry as 'not so much factories, but something like insurance company offices', as one official put it. Like others before it, the microchip industry was racing to limit the damage. 'We're taking all the precautions we know how to,' said a spokesman for the

Signetics Corporation, part of the Philips Group. 'Beyond going out of business, we don't know what else we can do.' However, he warned, 'a key question is that there still may be chemicals in use we don't know enough about, and that may be more harmful than we know. We're still learning. Even consultants in the field aren't sure how these things react.'

A surprisingly frank admission. No one expects that Silicon Valley will shut down while it cleans up its operations, but Chemie Linz, which ran the last plant in Europe manufacturing the herbicide 2,4,5-T and was the target of an anti-dioxin campaign, did just that, halting production of 2,4,5-T until it could develop a dioxin-free production route. Another German company, Boehringer Ingelheim, has also been forced to close a factory near Hamburg, following allegations that its dioxin-contaminated emissions had been responsible for birth defects (including cases of spina bifida and hydrocephalus) in the eastern part of Hamburg. Dioxin has often been seen as the ultimate toxin. Ranked as the most potent carcinogen by the US Environmental Protection Agency's cancer experts, it was thought to be about 100 million times as carcinogenic as a material such as vinyl chloride, which the EPA had restricted.

'Hardly a day goes by without some frightening headline about dioxin – or, more precisely, 2,3,7,8-tetrachlorodibenzo-p-dioxin, one of 75 dioxins,' the *Wall Street Journal* commented in a leader. 'This is reported to be the most toxic chemical made by man. Its presence in drainage ditches was one of the principal reasons families near Love Canal abandoned their homes. Europeans have just ended a search for some lost in transit. The US government bought out the town of Times Beach, Missouri, after the Centers for Disease Control recommended evacuation at exposures of more than one part per billion in soil samples. Traces of the toxin have been found in fish. And more than 16,000 Vietnam veterans have filed disability claims attributing skin disease, baldness, impotence, cancer and their children's birth defects to the dioxin in the defoliant Agent Orange.'

The reference to the 'lost dioxin' in Europe related to the intensive hunt for forty-one barrels of dioxin-contaminated waste which were part of the fallout from the explosion at Givaudan's Icmesa plant in Seveso. Hoffman-La Roche had consigned the barrels to Mannesmann, a West German company, for ultimate disposal. When it was realized that the wastes had not been incinerated as expected, the hunt was on. The barrels finally turned up in a disused abattoir in the village of Anguilcourt-le-Sart, near Saint-Quentin in France. As Givaudan's parent company, Hoffman-La Roche was exposed to a great deal of highly unwelcome publicity, although in the aftermath of the disaster the company had been the first into the field with chemical survey teams, mapping the distribution of the dioxin and collecting toxicological information. Unfortunately, it had taken five days before anyone realized that there had been dioxin in the cloud and eight days before local doctors were alerted. Local children had gaily played in the flakes of 'snow' which fell from the cloud and which were, it was discovered, almost pure dioxin.

Plants and animals were the first casualties. More than 700 people were eventually evacuated from Seveso, after protracted squabbles between the town authorities, the company and the government. Over 180 people contracted chloracne, a severe form of acne which can last for months, even years. The human health impact of the explosion is still unclear, but the confusion which reigned after the disaster led ninety women to have abortions, in case their exposure to dioxin had caused birth defects in the foetuses they were carrying at the time. Yet when German pathologists examined thirty of the aborted foetuses, they found that twenty-nine were normal, the thirtieth being too badly damaged for a reliable assessment to be made.

Chloracne was the only health problem conclusively attributed to the Seveso explosion by the time five Icmesa men received prison sentences of up to five years in 1983. They included the chairman of Icmesa and the plant's designer, technical director and engineering manager. Hoffman-La Roche, which had already paid out £80 million in compensation, was appalled by the court's judgement that the disaster could have been avoided. The 1976 explosion, it argued, had happened because a chemical reaction designed to produce trichlorophenol had been left unfinished in the reactor. The chemicals heated up spontaneously, the reactor having been switched off before the workforce went home for the weekend, and the resulting pressure blew out the safety valves. But, the companies said, a theory explaining this spontaneous reaction had only emerged five years after the explosion.

It had been far easier to prove negligence against the waste disposal contractor Russell Bliss, who contaminated a number of Missouri towns with dioxin. 'You could have told me it was some kind of new jelly and I'd have put it on toast and eaten it,' said Mr Bliss, after the event. What he had in fact done was to contract with a plant which made Agent Orange to dispose of by-product dioxin, mixing it with oil and spraying it on roads and in stable yards throughout the state. The mixture was meant to keep the dust down – and Mr Bliss was delighted to note that it kept the flies down too. Later, however, birds, cats and horses started to die. But the authorities were very slow to spot the emerging problem.

A stable owner filed suit against Mr Bliss in 1972, and his evidence mentioned that the streets of Times Beach had also been sprayed; but dioxin was still very much an unknown quantity, so no one took much notice. Some of the contaminated soil which was scraped from the stables was used as landfill for new houses in the town of Imperial. By 1974, the authorities had made the link between dioxin and animal deaths from cancer and liver disorders. They suggested that tests should be carried out in Imperial. When the EPA finally got round to conducting the tests, it found that the dioxin level was 300 parts per billion, at a time when the government considered as hazardous anything above one part per billion. Later the investigators tested Times Beach, and found 100 parts of dioxin per billion. Again, no one was sure what to do, until Nature took a hand. The Meramec river burst its banks later in the year, flooding Times Beach and carrying the dioxin into homes and shops. The EPA, after some further dithering, announced that the town would have to be evacuated.

'We believe that about 160 pounds of dioxin have been generated in the environment from this one factory,' said Fred Lafser, director of Missouri's Department of Natural Resources, 'and we still have between 30 and 40 pounds to trace.' The effect on the town's people was profound. 'The tension became unbearable,' said one woman. 'If we were exotic animals, the government would have protected us, but we are not an endangered species; so we've been ignored. The sense of depression is overwhelming.'

Indeed, the psychological impact of such a disaster may cause some of the ill-health later attributed to the spilled chemical. 'It's like living under the sword of Damocles,' said a psychologist who had studied a number of similar incidents. 'These people walk around with the feeling that there is a time bomb within them.' Among the side-effects of such stress, he noted, were loss of sleep, lack of appetite, headaches, heart palpitations, ulcers, failure of the immune response and even cancer.

The company which has been worst hit by the long-running dioxin controversy is Dow Chemical, second only to Du Pont in size in the United States and ranking sixth in most listings of the world's chemical companies in the early 1980s. 'Will the consumer buy a Dow kitchen cleaner if he thinks that Dow pollutes the environment with chemicals that give people cancer?' asked one Dow executive. 'Would you?' The question had become much more pressing because, while the company had been able to shrug off environmental pressure during the period when its income was rising consistently, its operating income slipped by a third between 1979 and 1982. Worse, Dow saw that the future lay in the speciality chemical market, rather than in bulk chemicals, hence the question. Whereas bulk chemicals are bought by small numbers of high-volume consumers, with the main concern being the price, speciality chemicals are bought by large numbers of small-volume consumers. Sometimes, in the form of cleaners or other household products, they are bought by individual consumers – who may find unacceptable the idea of buying something with the name Dow on the bottle or label.

At the time, Dow was a defendant in a suit filed by thousands of Vietnam veterans who had been exposed to Agent Orange, one ingredient of which was 2,4,5-T manufactured by Dow and others. Ever since 1897, when the company's founder, Herbert H. Dow, drilled down into brine pools below the plains around Midland searching for bromine, Dow has combined an emphasis on scientific excellence with an aggressive impatience with those it views as amateurs, particularly in the environmental field. 'We play our cards close,' admitted the company's chairman, Robert W. Lundeen, 'maybe because we have a high regard for the value of technical information. We don't back down easily or compromise. We are perceived as prickly, difficult, and arrogant.' That was to put it mildly.

As part of an attempt to rebuild its public image, Dow pulled five senior executives out from their normal duties to form an environmental action team. The company also paid out $3 million for a series of independent studies of the most serious allegations made against it. 'I have to say I was against it,' said company president Paul F. Oreffice. 'It smacks to me of trying to buy people off. But if we say we know the facts on something, we are accused of being arrogant. If we say we don't know all the answers, people say "You are killing people and you don't know the answers?" To be guilty until being proved innocent is ridiculous, but it is something we have to learn to live with.'

Critics accept that the company's science is excellent, and admit that its environmental performance is better than many of its competitors, but they fault Dow for downplaying the risks associated with toxic chemicals, its opposition to new regulations and other controls, and its readiness to take its opponents to court at the drop of a hat. A senior Dow toxicologist, for example, argued in testimony to Congress that dioxin had 'only mild effects' on people, whatever the animal tests might suggest. Although dioxin causes genetic changes, cancer and other chronic diseases in test animals, Dow has argued that we seem to be a resistant species.

The fatal dosage is certainly remarkably different in the various species of test animal: for example, it is 5,000 times as toxic in guinea pigs as in hamsters. On the human health front, Dow points to the first major dioxin accident, which happened in 1949 in Nitro, West Virginia, at a Monsanto plant that was producing 2,4,5-T. This release resulted in 121 workers developing chloracne and other symptoms. These workers were then studied over a period of thirty years – the University of Cincinnati's Institute of Environmental Health reported that the death rate in the group was lower than average while the frequency of cancers and other chronic diseases was either normal or below normal. Partly this may be due to the fact that those employed in the chemical industry generally tend to get better medical treatment than the average individual, but the result was none the less surprising for those who believed that the inevitable outcome of exposure to dioxin would be a burst of cancers and other serious diseases.

Other studies have suggested that there has been a significant rise in soft-tissue sarcomas, although the problem is that none of those suffering from such cancers have been exposed to dioxin alone, since dioxin, as a by-product, is never produced alone. Characteristically, Dow campaigned for the lifting of a 1979 ban on 2,4,5-T sales, despite the fact that the product was far from critical as far as future profits were concerned. But, the company explained, the ban 'was patently unsound and had no scientific merit. If we caved in on this one, we might lose the next one, when it was important.' In the end Dow did cave in, announcing that it would no longer make 2,4,5-T for the US market.

Dow's toxicology laboratory, founded in 1933, had pioneered the monitoring of toxic chemicals, developing instruments able to detect some of them at levels of a few parts per *quadrillion* – a few parts in a million billion. When the EPA found traces of forty toxic chemicals, including dioxin, in the effluent from Dow's Midland plant, Oreffice told shareholders that the level found, 50 parts per quadrillion, was equal to less than twenty drops in the plant's total annual discharge of 9 billion gallons into the Tittabawassee river.

Unfortunately such statistics have failed to reassure many of the company's critics. They point out that fish caged at the mouth of the plant's outlet accumulated 100 parts per trillion of dioxin, which was twice the level which the Food and Drug Administration had declared safe for consumption. Nor are they impressed with the company's achievements in cutting pollution generally. In fact, like 3M and other forward-thinking chemical companies, Dow has made major strides in this area, by switching production processes, recycling wastes and burning flammable gases in energy recovery plants. In 1960, for example, Dow produced a pound of waste for every pound of product, whereas by the early 1980s that balance had improved to a pound of waste for 1,000 pounds of product.

But Dow has remained under a glare of public scrutiny. Early in 1984 the authorities in the northern Brazilian state of Pará were exhuming foetuses, children and adults thought to have died because of the application of Dow's Tordon herbicides – which were a component of Agent Orange. The herbicides had been used to clear vegetation from the route of high-voltage power lines, over a distance of some 130 miles. The deaths, and a spate of miscarriages and malformed foetuses, were attributed by the state forensic team to the repeated sprayings.

Dow reacted in the usual way. Ruth Anderson of the company's UK subsidiary wrote to the *Financial Times* explaining that 'these herbicides are classified as low to moderate in toxicity. For example, the acute oral toxicity of Tordon 101 is comparable to the toxicity of table salt. Put into layman's terms, a person weighing 60 kg would have to drink more than 15 litres (4 gallons) of the actual Tordon 101 spray mixture to reach the oral acute LD_{50} level. Exposure of this magnitude or anything even remotely close to it would be impossible to achieve in actual use.'

But even Dow admits the herbicides may have been abused by those who applied them. News leaking out from the area suggested that the teams spraying the rights of way often washed their equipment in rivers used by local people for drinking water and washing purposes. And local women apparently used discarded herbicide drums for storing water and flour. Another possibility raised by local environmentalists, based on reports that the spray teams were adding powders to the spray mixture, is that someone had been experimenting with a new pesticide designed to clear the Amazon rain-forest. Paulo Nogueira Neto, head of the federal government's Environmental Secretariat, was so concerned that he sent samples of a white powder local people say was added to spray mixtures to Sweden and Finland for further analysis.

A company's scientific reputation is critically important if it is to operate effectively and safely at the toxic frontier, a fact of which Dow now needs no convincing. A related company, Dow Corning, has been trying for a long time to persuade regulators that its organosilicon products are the chemical equivalent of an innocent prisoner. The listing of all organosilicons on the 'black' or 'grey' lists of the various international marine pollution conventions, argued Jeffrey Raum of Dow Corning Europe, represents an 'un-justified innuendo against one of the safest classes of substances ever made by man'. Indeed, he has argued, their listing makes it less likely that they will be used in environmentally desirable applications, as in replacing PCBs in transformers. To date, the company says, some 15,000 transformers use organosilicon fluids compared to the 200,000 worldwide for which alternatives to PCBs must be found.

The original listing apparently happened because a single Dutch scientist expressed concern about the entire family of chemicals at a time when, in 1972, negotiations on the Oslo Convention on marine dumping of waste were being pushed forward rapidly in the wake of a dumping incident. They were listed because they are highly stable, like DDT and PCBs, and one particular family member (the phenyl silatranes) had proved toxic. But phenyl sila-tranes are mainly laboratory curiosities, and the only attempt to market them as pesticides had been based on their rapid break-down in water into harmless by-products.

The three main triggers for the listing of a class of chemical compounds on the 'black' or 'grey' lists are toxicity, persistence and bio-accumulation. Dow Corning is convinced that the most significant commercial organosilicons, including polymethylsil-oxane which accounts for about 90 per cent of all organosilicon production, are simply not toxic. And, as the company's ecologists stress, the fact that these compounds may be persistent does not mean that they should be likened to chlorinated hydrocarbons – they are not toxic to animals and do not bio-accumulate. The only slight concern is that Belgian scientists working for Dow Corning, who found no significant ecological effects, reported that the digestive processes of aquatic polyps were being slowed because prey species coated with high concentrations of polydimethylsiloxane appeared to be less accessible to their digestive enzymes.

The need for scientific integrity in coping with the succession of environmental issues which have buzzed around the chemical industry like a swarm of bees was also recognized at an early stage by Alan Robertson of ICI, who was instrumental in setting up the European Chemical Industry Ecology and Toxicology Centre (ECETOC). 'The big argument,' as Dr Robertson put it, 'is that we have in our 42 member companies the biggest resource, both in toxicology and ecology, in the world. Any government organization would be off its head if it didn't at least consult with us.'

Just as multinational regulatory agencies have had problems in trying to harmonize the legislation of their member states, so ECETOC had problems in building a consensus on how it should approach issues. 'We managed to get these companies together – and it wasn't easy,' Dr Robertson explained. 'I have great sympathy for the Secretary-General of the United Nations. There were ten different nationalities in that lot and none of them had exactly the same philosophy in the environmental field.' Inevitably, another problem has been to get those companies which are funding ECETOC's work to accept that the last thing it can afford to do is to whitewash one of its member's products. 'It's inevitable that if you are interested in toxicology or ecology,' Robertson continued, 'you find new truths which are damaging to business interests and some groups will say: Wait! That's not going to do us any good at all. But I said, look, as far as I am concerned, the first time you inhibit ECETOC on a research project or publication you can count on my resigning the next day. We can only influence governments, influence people and influence pressure groups if our scientific integrity is 100 per cent.'

Even with all this carefully husbanded integrity, the best that industry will sometimes be able to do is to say: We don't know what the answer is. We're still learning. In some instances we have the results of exhaustive animal tests, and we're running tests on many of the other potentially toxic chemicals. But we're still not entirely sure what some of those test results mean. We don't know, for example, whether the fact that a particular species of test animal develops a cancer or produces deformed offspring means that people will also do so, or whether the fact that all tests in animals have cleared a particular chemical means that it will be absolutely safe when people use it or are otherwise exposed to it.

Most of us would accept that we should subject such chemicals to animal tests before permitting them to be tried out on people – or on the foetal 'canaries' discussed earlier. But such tests can never guarantee safety and a growing number of people also believe that animal tests are an evil which no civilized society should tolerate. We have seen that new generations of 'electronic canary' have been developed, enabling us to detect astonishingly low concentrations of pollution, but they still cannot beat the living version in some applications. By law, every British colliery has to keep two canaries at the pithead, for use by mine rescue teams. The first whiff of carbon monoxide topples them from their perches, at which point they are taken back to the surface and, if they do not recover spontaneously, revived with a puff of oxygen. Computer-based sensors are also used but, as one mining official put it, 'They will not do the work as quickly or reliably as a canary. The canary's reaction is quick, certain and 100 per cent reliable.'

It would be nice to be able to say the same about animal toxicity tests. None the less, the close observation of wildlife has become a vital element in environmental protection, as is well illustrated by research carried out around Love Canal by John Christian of the State University of New York. He trapped field mice in three areas: along the fence immediately surrounding the toxic waste dump, the 'inner ring' which was evacuated in 1978; in the 'outer ring' where evacuation was optional; and 1.5 kilometres away where a control group was trapped. The age of the mice was calculated by weighing the lenses of their eyes and it was found that thirty-day-old mice in the control group lived for an average of a hundred days after trapping. Mice from the outer ring lived only seventy-five days on average and those unfortunates caught in the inner ring lasted a mere fifty-four days. Samples of fat taken from all three groups showed dichlorobenzene and polychlorinated biphenyls, while mice from the inner and outer rings were also contaminated with the pesticide Lindane (hexachlorocyclohexane) and 2-chlormethylnaphthene.

Some species seem to have been almost tailor-made to help us monitor pollution. A number of West German towns are using the elephant-trunk fish (*Gnathonemus petersi*), as was Bayer when I visited its Brunsbuettel production site. The fish normally emits 400 to 800 millisecond bursts a minute from its electric organs, designed to help it 'see' in murky water. But once expose these fish to water in which there is as little as 0.3 milligrams of lead per litre, or one part per 10,000 of trichloroethylene, and the frequency of their signals drops sharply. This change can be used to trigger an alarm system automatically, a distinct improvement on the old systems based on observing the behaviour of shrimp or trout.

The idea behind such systems, of course, is to keep the fish alive, in contrast to animal toxicity testing. A total of over 4 million animals were used in toxicity testing in the United Kingdom during 1982, down from a peak of 5.5 million in the mid-1970s. Of these, 80 per cent were rats and mice, 6 per cent were birds, and rabbits. Guinea pigs and fish accounted for a further 4 per cent each. The slaughter in the United States is even greater, with more than 60 million animals killed each year for experimental purposes in research laboratories, medical schools, colleges, and chemical and drug company research facilities. Some 30 million of these are rodents, and other, more controversial, victims include over 160,000 dogs, 50,000 cats and 47,000 monkeys.

Many of these animals are bred for the purpose, but pet-lovers in North America have protested against the use of discarded pet dogs. Conservationists, too, are increasingly (and justifiably) alarmed by the way that monkeys and other primates are being stripped out of the tropical rain-forests, themselves endangered, for use in laboratory experiments. Faced with tightening restrictions on the export of some primates, for example chimpanzees, companies like Immuno have set up research facilities in such countries as Sierra Leone to ensure direct access to animals taken from the wild. The damage caused by this traffic is suggested by the fact that the only way to capture wild chimps is to kill the mothers and take the infants. Such projects will ultimately prove unsustainable, either because they exhaust the wild populations or because of pressure from the World Health Organisation, which specifies that endangered, rare or vulnerable animals should only be taken from 'existing, self-sustaining breeding colonies'.

'What really stopped human slavery was the growth of the

industrial society and the need for humans as purchasers rather than as slaves,' says Cyril Rosen, UK secretary of the International Primate Protection League. 'If monkeys become so scarce and expensive that they are an impractical tool for much routine work – as is becoming the case – then the alternative is to look for cheaper tools. Man is ingenious enough to find those other means.'

Animal tests have many advantages as far as the tester is concerned. The rabbit's eye, for example, tends to be sensitive to most of the things that the human eye is sensitive to. Its tear ducts are relatively undeveloped, so that the irritant you introduce stays there longer; and the resulting inflammation shows up nicely on the rabbit's unpigmented eye. This, the Draize test, has been the target of a carefully focused US campaign since Henry Spira welded nearly 400 groups into an anti-Draize coalition. Another main target has been the acute oral toxicity test, with the LD_{50} test, which is being written into one piece of legislation after another around the world, generally being seen as the villain of the piece.

The LD_{50} test, as we have seen, is meant to establish the short-term effect of a single dose of a suspected toxin, and accounts for a great many animals. Used in the safety testing of drugs, food additives, agricultural chemicals and a wide range of consumer products, the LD_{50} test is generally carried out on rats, mice and either rabbits or dogs – or both. While the tests leave a considerable number of animals poisoned to a greater or lesser degree, they are not good at telling us what we need to know. One of the leading proponents of alternative, non-animal testing methods, the Fund for the Replacement of Animals in Medical Experiments (FRAME), insists that 'the use of large numbers of animals to meet the needs of statistical analysis satisfies bureaucratic rather than scientific requirements'. This view is supported by a growing number of scientists, who see the LD_{50} test as reducing toxicology from an exercise of reasoned intellect to a mechanical operation often serving no good purpose.

Worse, there is the central problem that different species react in different ways, which FRAME believes 'makes a mockery of the accurate determination of an LD_{50} for a rodent, rabbit or dog with the intention of extrapolating the figure to man'. The LD_{50} test aims to determine the dose of a toxin which will kill 50 per cent of the animals to which it is fed, yet the LD_{50} values for a chemical like methylfluoroacetate range from 0.15 in mice to 11.0 in monkeys, with an estimated value for human victims of 3.85.

The test has the virtue of simplicity, however: a substance can be categorized as harmful if the LD_{50} for an oral dose is around 500 milligrams per kilogram of body-weight, toxic if the LD_{50} is 50 mg and very toxic if it is 5 mg. And new LD_{50} procedures are being developed, with toxicologists such as Michael van der Heuval convinced that they can produce better science with less suffering and death among laboratory animals.

Apart from the problems revolving around the availability and reliability of laboratory animals, there has been the growing cost of simply keeping them housed and fed to the standards now required. Coupled with the increasing public hostility to animal tests in many countries, these factors have contributed to a significant softening of industrial attitudes. In 1980 Revlon gave Rockefeller University $750,000 to help it identify and develop alternatives to the Draize test, and even larger grants have since been donated by industry to research teams developing non-animal tests. This investment is beginning to pay off, with researchers at Tufts University growing human cornea cells as an alternative to the Draize test, an alternative which they expect to be both cheaper and more effective. In Britain, too, research into alternatives is booming. In the Department of Clinical Pharmacology at St Bartholomew's Hospital, for example, tests have shown that human sperm can be used as an extremely sensitive indicator of the local anaesthetic activity of beta-blockers, drugs which are used in the treatment of heart disease – research which has suggested the possibility of using beta-blockers as a male contraceptive. Another approach involves using the human placenta itself to test new drugs. Researchers at London's Charing Cross Hospital, for example, have developed a new way of maintaining human placentas received just minutes after birth for use in reproductive toxicity tests.

One of the most hopeful research programmes was launched in 1982 by FRAME, with £250,000 from industrial sponsors such as Avon Cosmetics, Bristol-Myers, Hoechst UK, Johnson & Johnson, Pfizer, and Rimmel International. Although the ultimate objective of FRAME's research is to achieve the complete replacement of animal experiments by 'scientifically valid and economically acceptable alternatives', it is convinced that the transition can be achieved only in carefully orchestrated stages.

Defining 'alternative' tests as including any technique that replaces or reduces the use of animals in biomedical experiments, FRAME distinguishes between (and supports) four main categories of alternative research: the use of micro-organisms and lower vertebrates; cell, tissue or organ culture; mathematical and computer models; and human and epidemiological studies. The most enormous ingenuity is going into the development of computer models which can sound an early alarm on the basis of analysing a compound atom by atom, and cross-checking its structure with other compounds known to cause problems. The same computer programmes can be used to work backwards, using information about an observed side-effect, such as a tendency for a rat's tail to go rigid, to pinpoint the chemical which is responsible.

Unfortunately, such models are not yet much use for reliably spotting carcinogens, mutagens or teratogens. Indeed, FRAME has admitted that 'the complex nature of the reproductive process, the multiple processes involved in gametogenesis, fertilization, implantation and embryonic development, and the three metabolic "compartments" involved (the mother, placenta and foetus) make accurate experimental modelling difficult, particularly when inter-species differences act as further confounding factors. As yet,' it cautions, 'there is no alternative to the use of whole animals in reproductive toxicity testing.'

Most countries are now insisting on a battery of tests, starting with bacterial systems and progressively working up through cell, tissue and organ culture to clinical trials on human volunteers and full-scale epidemiological studies once the cleared product is in wide use. The expense involved can be very considerable, and the efforts of conservative administrations to cut back on their expenditure in the fields of health, safety and environment should have come as no surprise. Similarly, the sacking of some of the Environmental Protection Agency's best scientists (on the grounds that they were 'bleeding-heart liberals', 'poison' or 'invidious environmental extremists', as the EPA hit-list described them) was only to be expected. But today's industrial societies continue to push through the 'toxic frontier' of our current understanding of toxicology. Like experimental rats in a laboratory maze, they need all their faculties to ensure that they negotiate their way through this highly complicated, and on occasions extremely dangerous, environment. Purging your critical scientists and toxicologists is rather like giving your experimental rat a frontal lobotomy. Consider what might have happened, for example, if Dr Kelsey

(p. 101) had been sacked before the thalidomide problem emerged.

'People in a free society are at liberty to take certain risks,' said Arthur Upton, former director of the US National Cancer Institute, reacting to the cuts imposed by the Reagan administration. 'The regulator has to have a sense of what the society wants in terms of restriction and fit the scientific evidence into the equation. What worries me is that the present administration seems to be going beyond a wholesome and reasonable reassessment of the evidence.'

Indeed, before long this approach had backfired seriously on the Reagan administration. Among the problems which surfaced was the controversy about ethylene dibromide (EDB), which animal tests carried out at the US National Cancer Institute and elsewhere showed can cause sterility, birth defects and cancer. This pesticide, also known as dibromoethane, is structurally similar to dibromo-chloropropane (DBCP) and has been used as a fumigant in grain milling and storage and in citrus fruit production. It is also used in leaded fuels to prevent the build-up of lead in car engines. Some 300 million pounds of EDB were manufactured in the USA during 1983, with Dow Chemical estimating that 90 per cent went into gasoline, with the rest injected into soil or sprayed on crops.

Shortly before Christmas of 1983, health and agricultural officials in Florida found traces of EDB in a whole range of grain-based foods, triggering an astonishing uproar among consumers. The Environmental Protection Agency published figures suggesting that 50 to 70 per cent of the nation's grain stockpile contained measurable levels of EDB.

Under President Carter, the EPA had proposed a ban on EDB in many applications, but the incoming Republican administration had called a meeting of food industry representatives at the White House and, with Mrs Gorsuch then in control of the EPA, the regulatory programme had been dropped. And the devolution of environmental controls from federal to state agencies compounded the eventual crisis, with individual states setting widely different standards for EDB concentrations in food. 'We believe there is no safe level for a carcinogen,' said Massachusetts Public Health Commissioner Bailus Walker Jr. Massachusetts voted for an immediate ban on the sale of all food products containing 10 parts per billion or more of EDB – and warned that products containing a single part per billion would soon be ordered off the shelves.

Taken completely by surprise, the US food industry set up the

American Grain Products Processing Institute to put across the
other side of the story – but the damage had already been done.
Once again, a major industry had been caught unawares by public
concerns about the safety of its products.

Ultimately, life is a risky business and people will have to learn
to make some very difficult trade-offs. No one believes that cancer
victims should turn down treatment, but it is increasingly clear
that some of the drug and radiation therapies used are themselves
causing cancer. 'It's fairly common to see patients on these kinds
of treatment developing leukaemia a few years down the line,'
explained John Boice, one of the authors of a study which showed
that, of 2,067 patients studied, fourteen developed leukaemia
during a six-year period compared to only one individual in a
1,566-person control group. Most of us would see that risk as well
worth running.

But what about isotrietinoin, marketed by Hoffman-La Roche as
Roaccutane in Britain and Accutane in the United States? The drug
is used to treat severe acne, and animal tests have clearly shown
its key ingredient, a derivative of vitamin A, to be teratogenic.
Despite this evidence, it was decided that the drug's benefits out-
weighed any negative aspects, and Hoffman-La Roche was then
faced with a small number of cases of women who had taken the
drug during pregnancy and subsequently had either suffered
spontaneous abortions or given birth to children with serious brain
deformities. A spokesman for the US Food and Drug Administration said that the company was not to blame. 'You can't ensure
that patients will do what they're told,' she said. 'There are quite
a number of drugs on the market that are teratogenic,' she added,
'and it's not entirely unusual to have to depend on the health
profession to inform patients of the risk.' In the wake of the problems, however, Hoffman-La Roche made its warnings much more
visible on the packs and recommended that women patients should
not become pregnant for at least a month after their treatment had
ended.

Even thalidomide, which gave an enormous boost to reproductive toxicology around the world, is back in use, with great care
being taken to ensure that any patients fully understand the risk
and avoid pregnancy during treatment for Behçet's syndrome.
Later on, it may also be used to treat severe rheumatoid arthritis.
'One really has to use this drug,' said one of the consultants
involved, 'because these patients do not respond to other treatment

and their lives are such a misery. One woman whom we treated last year said that last Christmas was the first she had looked forward to for eight years. It has no complications in the non-pregnant, other than possible tingling in the hands and feet of some patients.'

Where drugs adversely affect only a small number of those treated, the attention may switch to screening them out at an early stage. 'I think we are going to find many more genetic defects and many more drugs which are affected,' is the way that Professor Robert Smith of St Mary's Hospital Medical School, London, put it. 'And I think this is the beginning of a new way of looking at drugs and how they should be prescribed. Until now adverse reactions were generally blamed on the drug. I think from now on we will be looking far more at the individual and how he or she handles the drug.' Professor Smith had himself proved unusually sensitive to the drug debrisoquine, and estimated that five million Britons, or one person in ten, has a genetic defect which could cause them to react badly to at least one drug.

Even new products which have successfully passed all the tests in animals and human volunteers can hit problems once in wide use because of the genetic diversity in every community (described Chapter 8). Take aspartame, marketed as a safer and tastier substitute for saccharin. It soon emerged that a considerable number of people who suffer from an inherited inability to metabolize one of aspartame's two main ingredients, phenylalinine, could be at risk. In the United States an estimated four million people have a genetic predisposition to this condition, known as phenyl-ketonuria, with a further one million in Britain. The most serious effects are likely to be seen in pregnant women, given that women with raised phenylalinine levels are at a greater risk of producing babies with such defects as microcephaly, mental retardation and other neurological disorders.

Having spent over £160 million on developing and marketing aspartame, manufacturers G. D. Searle are unlikely to want to withdraw it, although patients known to have phenylketonuria have been warned of the danger in Britain. 'The quantity of aspartame in soft drinks causes brain levels of phenylalinine the like of which has never occurred in man's evolutionary history,' warned Professor Robert Wurtman of the Massachusetts Institute of Technology (MIT). 'It's going to be a fascinating experiment in brain chemistry. Do we really want to conduct this experiment?'

The fact remains that we are the ultimate experimental animal. We invent and manufacture mind-numbing numbers of chemical and other products and will presumably continue to do so. At the same time, we have turned our world into a planetary laboratory in which we are rapidly becoming the key test organism. Many of the things we do have an effect on our life expectancy and our health in later life. But we are also, unfortunately, hopeless experimental animals, exposing ourselves wittingly or unwittingly to an enormous number of factors which may affect the ultimate outcome. Epidemiologists, who study the links between exposure and health, have a desperately hard time of it. 'Few hazards have been subject to more detailed epidemiological evaluation than cigarette smoking and exposure to ionising radiation or asbestos,' the Royal Society noted, 'but for none do we yet know whether there are thresholds at very low levels (e.g. the smoke of other people's cigarettes), nor do we have established dose-response relationships.'

At least if we are dealing with a group of people who have been exposed to asbestos or ionizing radiation, we know roughly what we are looking for. We also know where and when we might see it. But reproductive toxicology can be a far trickier area. Take smoking as an example. There are many ways in which smoking can affect the health of the unborn, but not all of them are necessarily disadvantageous. We started this journey through reproductive toxicology in the company of a young Japanese mother-to-be. In the normal course of events we would expect her baby to be smaller than normal because of her smoking, apart from any other problems which might be discovered at a later date. But research carried out at the Sergievsky Center at Columbia University, New York, suggests that her smoking could actually cut her baby's risks of trisomy, which involves the presence of an extra chromosome and can lead to such disorders as Down's syndrome. Jennie Kline and her colleagues knew that up to 97 per cent of embryos with autosomal trisomies abort spontaneously by the seventeenth week of gestation. They also knew that no environmental agent had previously been conclusively shown to be associated with the frequency of trisomy, so they were surprised to find that their research results showed that, while older women who smoked around the time of conception were running an even higher risk of having children affected by trisomy, younger women actually appeared to be reducing that risk by smoking around the time of conception.

No one doubts that on balance smoking is harmful to the unborn, but this example does illustrate the complexity of the systems with which we are dealing. Of course, our reproductive systems have been under environmental challenge since we began to evolve on this planet, and many naturally occurring substances continue to disrupt reproduction. Cassava, which is a staple food for millions of people in Africa, Asia and South America, has now been shown to cause birth defects if eaten in large quantities by mothers-to-be. Researchers at the University of Calabar, Nigeria, found that laboratory rats fed with cassava powder as 50 or 80 per cent of their diet during the first fifteen days of pregnancy showed a range of health effects. Because of the low protein content of cassava, the birthweight of babies born to cassava-fed rats was considerably less than the birthweight of those born to control group mothers, and a high proportion of deformed offspring were produced by the cassava-fed rats. Of the embryos implanted in the uterus, 19 per cent died at a very early stage and were resorbed, while 28 per cent showed such abnormalities as limb defects and malformations of the eye and brain. The root cause of the problems was thought to be cyanide, with every 100 grams of cassava releasing 0.1 to 2 milligrams of cyanide when exposed to the enzyme hydrolase. The cyanide appeared to poison the nervous system, very much like thalidomide, and interrupted the differentiation of limbs in the embryo.

But Rachel Carson's central thesis still holds true: the chemicals likely to cause the greatest damage to our reproductive systems and to which the greatest number of people around the world are exposed at one time or another are those used to protect crops. 'A scandal of global proportions' is the way David Weir and Mark Schapiro of the San Francisco-based Institute for Food and Development Policy described the international traffic in pesticides which had been banned or restricted in the developed and more environmentally sensitive countries. Their book, *Circle of Poison*, provided damning evidence that the decision of the Reagan administration to relax export controls on such pesticides was backfiring seriously. Used to spray crops in the developing world, the pesticides contaminated fruit and other crop products. Some of these were promptly re-exported to the United States and other major markets, like a chemical boomerang.

In a worrying study carried out by Britain's highly reputable

Association of Public Analysts, and reported in 1984 by the *Sunday Times*, one-third of all the fresh fruit and vegetables tested proved to be contaminated by chemical residues. Despite the fact that DDT is technically banned under a voluntary agreement between pesticide producers and the Ministry of Agriculture, the long-standing Pesticides Safety Precautions Scheme, DDT was found in 119 of 132 samples of apples, lettuce and mushrooms tested in a single day. Lindane, banned in the United States after it was shown to cause foetal cancer, is still used in Britain – and nineteen of a sample of thirty-seven pears were found to contain the pesticide. Lindane was also found in nearly half of a sample of strawberries, bought at random from shops around the country, as well as in aubergines, beans, cauliflowers, lettuce, mushrooms and tomatoes. The pressure for tighter, regulatory (rather than voluntary) controls led to the astonishing spectacle of Britain's pesticide industry joining environmentalists in lobbying *for* such controls, while Mrs Thatcher's Cabinet, with its strong links with the farming community, initially dragged its heels.

Despite the enormous increase in consumption of fresh fruit and vegetables, the British government has failed to fund the research needed to determine whether or not there is a real threat to health from the use of pesticides. The Institution of Environmental Health Officers has been lobbying for a central sampling scheme, a call supported by the British Medical Association – which represents the country's doctors.

Increasingly, development agencies and the various campaigning organizations are recognizing that environmental, health and development targets are inextricably linked. In helping to set up the Pesticides Action Network in 1982, Oxfam calculated that there were then some 750,000 pesticide poisonings around the world each year, with perhaps 375,000 of these occurring in the Third World – where a high proportion of the poisonings result from 'the availability, often with very little effective restriction or control, of very toxic pesticides in conditions where the necessary safety precautions are highly unrealistic'. Pesticides which have been restricted in the developed nations, including malathion, dieldrin, aldrin, DDT and gamma BHC, are freely available in the Third World, and are often sold with inadequate safety information.

In the wake of a number of ecological disasters, attributed to pesticide abuse, which had severely damaged Thailand's fish-breeding industry, a Thai toxic substances expert working in the Country's Agriculture Department explained that 'many chemicals banned in the developed countries are sold cheaply here. In some areas, people use chemicals which are formulated by local distributors and don't even have labels. They just mix two or three together like a cocktail. They just know that one is to kill insects and another is to kill weeds, but they don't know which insects or weeds, or how much the dosage should be.' And it is not just the wilder species of life which suffer: the illiterate farmers and farm labourers are often drenched and little is done to protect their livestock or families.

Some of the more reputable pesticide manufacturers have been trying hard to ensure that their performance is beyond reproach, but even companies such as Ciba-Geigy, which has called for fairer treatment for the agrochemical industry, have shown an unhappy knack for destroying their own case. Ciba-Geigy was acutely embarrassed when a Swiss TV programme uncovered evidence showing that it had intentionally sprayed unprotected Egyptian children with the insecticide Galecron. The objective was to see how much of the insecticide was excreted. Ciba-Geigy's European publicity for Galecron had stressed that children should be kept away from the insecticide, and the product was taken off the market for a period in 1976 after it was found that it increased tumour rates in laboratory mice. It was reintroduced later, but only for use on cotton, where it was particularly effective against pests which had become resistant to DDT.

'When life is often nasty, brutish and short,' the British Agrochemicals Association has said in defence of continuing British exports of problem pesticides to the Third World, 'the significance of a persistent organo-chlorine insecticide pales alongside the lives it can save.' True, as far as it goes. And it is also true that Rachel Carson's worst fears have not been realized, largely because of the enormous political backlash created by Silent Spring. But in a shrinking world we must develop much more intelligent approaches to the management of our environmental resources.

Rachel Carson talked about integrated pest management, which does not rely solely on pesticides, and major strides have been made in the field since she died. But there is a paradox here: integrated pest management requires, among other things, a number of highly specific pesticides, so that farmers can 'ring the changes' on pests, switching from one pesticide to another before the pest has time to build up resistance. But the cost of testing such chemicals for toxicity now means that it is difficult to justify their development for relatively small and specialized markets. And the same argument holds true in the medical field, where we see the phenomenon of 'orphan' drugs, capable of treating forms of disease affecting only relatively small numbers of people. The cost of testing them to today's standards would make them uneconomic.

This does not mean that pesticides, drugs and other products should not be subjected to such tests, but it does mean that we should do everything we can to ensure that any expense is necessary and gives us the return we need in the form of toxicological and ecological data. We still have a long way to go before we can hope to comprehend the long-term health and ecological effects of life on, or beyond, the toxic frontier.

'We're dealing with a science that's only two decades old,' cautions the director of the US National Toxicology Program, Dr David Rall. 'It's a baby compared to other biomedical sciences. I think we'll be in much better shape with the experience of another ten years.' In the meantime, we must accept that we are the ultimate experimental animal and act accordingly. If we have another Seveso or Love Canal, as India now has in Bhopal (see p. 11), we have to make sure that we extract as much information from the unplanned, unwanted experiment. The epidemiological work carried out in the aftermath of Seveso was severely handicapped. The background information on birth defects, miscarriages and liver malfunction was very poor, so it was difficult to decide what was a 'natural' background effect and what was an effect resulting from exposure to dioxin. The situation has improved in many parts of Europe, but the same problems would still face investigators in many parts of the world, particularly in the Third World. Another problem at Seveso was that, in the early years at least, the work was entrusted to nearby Milan University, which was by no stretch of the imagination a centre of excellence in toxicology. By the time the work was transferred elsewhere, the vital early years had passed and had not been adequately covered.

Or take the example of Triana, a small town in Alabama, whose mainly black and poor inhabitants were massively contaminated with DDT by a plant run by the Olin Corporation. The Redstone arsenal closed in 1971, but it was only in 1983 that the residents won a $19 million settlement from Olin, which also agreed to try to clean up the DDT within ten years and to monitor the health of those who had been exposed. The DDT-contaminated effluents from the plant had flowed right through the centre of town, in Indian Creek. DDT levels in five species of fish averaged over 200 parts per million, peaking at 405 ppm, while wildfowl in a nearby swamp proved to have up to 2,252 ppm of DDT in their flesh.

It took eight years for epidemiologists from the Centers for Disease Control in Atlanta, Georgia, to take samples of blood from Triana residents. In one case, the results showed a level of DDT twice as high as anything previously reported in the literature, while other results were comparable with those previously only seen in heavily exposed workers in DDT factories. An ideal opportunity, one would have thought, to study the long-term health effects of DDT; but the Centers for Disease Control focused on the ecological effects and pleaded budget cuts when it came to thinking about the long-term human health effects. It has also been claimed that the unusually uniform socio-economic status of Triana's poor black residents made it far from easy to identify a control group for comparison.

This is simply not good enough. When William Ruckelshaus was faced with one of his first major crises as EPA administrator, a crisis focusing on a massive copper-smelter operated by Asarco Inc., near Tacoma, Washington State, he observed that the only way he felt he could get a fair ruling was to 'open it clear up. Let every bit of information we have out, and let the public wrestle with it the same as we do.' But budget cuts may mean that the information is never produced. The problem in Tacoma was arsenic, which can cause cancer. Given that the eighty-acre plant pumped some $35 million a year into the local economy, critics felt that asking the community to decide on the plant's future was 'economic blackmail'. 'People,' it was felt, 'will vote for jobs and cancer.' Once again, as we saw happened in Brazil's Vila Parisi (see p. 21), people were being backed into a corner: the last thing they wanted was to be unemployed, but they certainly did not want their children developing cancer either. 'You're balancing money and lives,' said Richard Ayres, head of the US National Clean Air Coalition, 'and they just don't balance.'

Tragically, even the veritable epidemic of anencephaly cases reported around Cubatão paled beside the human toll of the fireball which swept through Vila Socó, a Cubatão favela housing some 9,000 people, on 25 February 1984. As highly inflammable gasoline leaked from a Petrobrás pipeline, opened in error, a fireball was ignited which reached 1,000°C and incinerated eight and a half acres of wooden shacks. Eighty-six bodies were counted, but Coroner Carlos Affonso Figueiredo thought it strange that no bodies of children under five had been found. It was then deduced that the fireball was so hot that, as Figueiredo put it, 'the bodies of young children trapped in the blaze were literally cremated. And since whole families were killed, there was no one to report the children's deaths or disappearance.'

Later it was calculated that probably more than 500 people perished in the disaster, including an estimated 300 children. Petrobrás, which had failed to notice that the irrigation ditches around the *favela* had filled with gasoline, turning the area into a huge potential incendiary bomb, said it would compensate the survivors. In many ways, as is often the case, an outright disaster provoked a response where a slowly emerging chronic health problem had been brushed under the political carpet. It is easier to prove that you have been caught in a fireball than that your child's anencephaly has been caused by industrial pollution.

It is far too early to know whether the Bhopal gas leak will produce any genetic effects. Indeed, at the time of writing it was also too soon to say whether there would be any birth defects among children born to female victims. An initial estimate was that at least 1,000 pregnant women were caught in the gas cloud. 'All the pregnant women are being followed up,' a spokesman at Bhopal's Mahatma Gandhi Medical College assured the press. 'We shall be checking for two years to see if there are any developmental or intelligence defects.'

Inevitably people are beginning to come up with methods for detoxifying other people. The Foundation for Advancements in Science and Education, based in Los Angeles, has tested the Hubbard detoxification programme on some of those exposed to polybrominated biphenyls after the Michigan disaster which left nine million people with PBBs in their tissues. The programme is based on carefully orchestrated exercise, sauna and dieting, with increasing doses of niacin to trigger the release of toxins from the tissues. The levels of toxin in the blood, fat and urine were monitored by gas chromatography and it was found that 25 per cent of the body's burden of toxins could be removed during a twenty-day programme. Interestingly, those treated in this way found that their reaction times improved by 20 per cent and their long-term memory by over 15 per cent.

Clearly this represents a significant potential breakthrough, but the inevitable question surfaces: should we ever have got to the stage where we have to decontaminate nearly nine million people? However you answer the question, the fact remains that we are no longer talking simply of wildlife, we are talking about us. When *Silent Spring* burst on a largely unsuspecting world, we were talking about the reproductive failures of animals and birds. Today we know that our sperm, our eggs, our embryos and our children are in the front line.

As a result we are seeing one of the most hopeful environmental trends for years, with a new grass-roots environmental movement springing up among the uncounted millions of the once silent majority who are not environmental activists, environmental scientists or environmental journalists. Whereas environmental protection has all too often been the preserve of the affluent or of those, such as students, who are outside the mainstream economy, this time round the movement is gathering from a different direction, from those who have suddenly become aware that they live or work along the toxic frontier.

'We're not dope-smoking, hippie environmentalists,' says a pharmacist from Lexington, Tennessee. A few years earlier he would almost certainly have helped run any 'environmentalist' out of town. Today, with a toxic waste disposal site proposed in his own home-town, he is fighting mad. Once, when environmentalists asked him to consider future generations, he found it hard. Now the argument has hit home: those future generations start with his own children. 'We're a new breed,' he asserts. 'We drive pick-up trucks and wear overalls. And we'll be much harder to stop.' We must hope so.

PRINCIPAL SOURCES

INTRODUCTION: MOTHER-TO-BE

p. 17 Clair C. Patterson, 'Natural Levels of Lead in Humans', California Institute of Technology, Division of Geological and Planetary Sciences, Pasadena, California 91125, USA

p. 18 Richard D. Lyons, 'Disabilities in US Babies Found to Have Doubled in 25 Years', *International Herald Tribune*, 31 July 1983

p. 19 Tracy Dahlby, 'Japan is Winning War on Pollution', *International Herald Tribune*, 25 March 1983. See also Jumpei Audo, 'Pollution Control in Japan', *Journal of Japanese Trade & Industry*, No. 5, 1983, pp. 12–14

Mario Shao, 'Taiwan Gets Rude Awakening to the Problems of Pollution', *Wall Street Journal*, 18 July 1983, p. 20

p. 21 Hunter R. Clark, 'No Stars in the "Valley of Death"', *Time*, 19 September 1983, pp. 46–7

p. 23 Catherine Caufield, 'Germans Come Clean on Titanium Dioxide Waste', *New Scientist*, 25 August 1983, p. 528

'Fish Cancer Found Widely in the US', *New Scientist*, 29 September 1983, p. 913

p. 25 Robin McKie, 'Windscale Dilemma: Is Radiation Ever Safe?', *Observer*, 6 November 1983, p. 2

p. 26 *Investigation of the Possible Increased Incidence of Cancer in West Cumbria* (the Black Report), Report of an Independent Advisory Group chaired by Sir Douglas Black, HMSO, London, 1984

1: ONE IN A TRILLION

p. 29 Masahiro Ochiai, Michiko Ohotomi, Yoshinari Ambe, Hiroyuki Shinohara and Takahisa Hanya, 'Secular Variation of BHC in the Paper of Books', *The Science of the Total Environment*, 5 (1976), pp. 273–6

p. 31 John R. Holum, *Topics and Terms in Environmental Problems*, Wiley Interscience, 1977, particularly pp. 379–83 and 456–60

The Global Environment Monitoring System, United Nations Environment Programme, UNEP, 1982

p. 32 D. Taylor, *Inorganic Mercury as a Contributory Factor in the Initial Outbreak of Minamata Disease in Japan*, ICI Brixham Laboratory Policy Briefing, BL/PB/6, January 1981

p. 34 Michael G. Petit and J. Scott Altenbach, 'A Chronological Record of Environmental Chemicals from Analysis of Stratified Vertebrate Excretion Deposited in a Sheltered Environment', *Environmental Research*, 6 (1973), pp. 339–43

p. 35 C. Tuthill, W. Schutte, C. W. Frank, J. Santolucito and G. Potter, 'Retrospective Monitoring: A Review', *Environmental Monitoring and Assessment*, 1 (1982), pp. 189–211

M. H. Martin and P. J. Coughtrey, *Biological Monitoring of Heavy Metal Pollution: Land and Air*, Applied Science, 1982, pp. 337–57

p. 36 David Jones, 'The Singular Case of Napoleon's Wallpaper', *New Scientist*, 14 October 1982, pp. 101–4

David E. H. Jones and Kenneth W. D. Ledingham, 'Arsenic in Napoleon's Wallpaper', *Nature*, Vol. 299, 14 October 1982, pp. 626–7

p. 40 Clair C. Patterson 'Mega-Exposures to Lead', *Lead Versus Health*, ed. M. Rutter and R. Russell Jones, John Wiley & Sons, 1983, pp. 17–32

p. 44 *Identifying and Estimating the Genetic Impact of Chemical Mutagens*, National Academy Press, 1983

p. 46 'Toxic Metals Go Down the Drain – and into the Drinking Water', *New Scientist*, 28 October 1982, p. 235

Rachel Carson, *Silent Spring*, Pelican Books, 1982. Originally published by Houghton Mifflin, 1962

2: THE ENDANGERED SPERM

p. 48 Eric Jansson, 'White Paper: The Impact of Hazardous Substances upon Infertility Among Men in the United States', Friends of the Earth, Washington, DC, 17 November 1980

pp. 50–51 W. H. James, 'Secular Trends in Reported Sperm Counts', *Andrologia*, 12 (1980), pp. 381–8

J. MacLeod and Y. Wang, 'Male Fertility Potential in Terms of Semen Quality: A Review of the Past, a Study of the Present', *Fertil. Steril.*, 31 (1979), pp. 103–16

p. 53 Arielle Emmett, 'The Sperm Scare', *The Weekly: Seattle's Newsmagazine*, 23 July 1980, p. 14

p. 54 Justin M. Joffe, 'Influence of Drug Exposure of the Father on Perinatal Outcome', Symposium on Pharmacology, *Clinics in Perinatology*, Vol. 6, No. 1, March 1979, pp. 21–36

p. 55 P. S. Weathersbee, L. K. Olsen and J. R. Lodge, 'Caffeine and

Pregnancy: A Retrospective Study', *Postgraduate Medicine*, Vol. 62, 1977, pp. 64–9

p. 58 S. M. Barlow and F. M. Sullivan, *Reproductive Hazards of Industrial Chemicals*, Academic Press, 1982, pp. 212–29

Robert J. Huggett and Michael E. Bender, 'Kepone in the James River', *Environmental Science & Technology*, August 1980, pp. 918–23

Marvin H. Zim, 'Allied Chemical's $20 Million Ordeal with Kepone', *Fortune*, 11 September 1978, pp. 82–91. See also Lisa Miller Mesdag, 'Remember Kepone?', *Fortune*, 22 August 1983, p. 193

3: UNBORN CANARIES

p. 65 Rachel Carson, *Silent Spring*, Pelican Books, 1982, pp. 36–8

p. 66 S. M. Barlow and F. M. Sullivan, op. cit., pp. v, 40

Ronald Bayer, 'Reproductive Hazards in the Workplace: Bearing the Burden of Fetal Risk', *Millbank Memorial Fund Quarterly/ Health and Society*, Vol. 60, No. 4, 1982, pp. 633–56

p. 67 *Interpretive Guidelines on Employment Discrimination and Reproductive Hazards*, in the *Federal Register*, Equal Employment Opportunity Commission and the Office of Federal Contracts Compliance Programs, 1 February 1980, p. 7514

p. 68 *Chemical Hazards to Human Reproduction*, Council on Environmental Quality, US Government Printing Office, 1981

p. 70 'Effects of Lead on Reproduction: Review of Experimental Studies', *Lead Versus Health*, ed. M. Rutter and R. Russell Jones, John Wiley & Sons, 1983, pp. 217–27

p. 71 R. B. McFarland and H. Reigel, 'Chronic Mercury Poisoning from a Single Brief Exposure', *Journal of Occupational Medicine*, Vol. 20, No. 8, 1978, pp. 532–4

p. 72 'Chronic Manganese Poisoning: Clinical Picture and Manganese Turnover', *Neurology*, Vol. 17, 1967, pp. 128–36

p. 73 'Importance of the Nutrition Factor in the Comprehensive Social Hygiene Study of the Health of Female Workers in the Chemical Industry', *Gigiena I. Sanitariya*, 1 (1979)

p. 74 A. V. Shumilina, 'Menstrual and Child-Bearing Functions of Female Workers Occupationally Exposed to the Effects of Formaldehyde', *Gigiena Truda I Professional 'Nye Zabolevaniya*, 12 (1975), pp. 18–21

Criteria Document for a Recommended Standard: Occupational Exposure to Chloroprene, US Department of Health, Education and Welfare/ NIOSH, Publication Nos. 77–210, 1977

Z. Panova and G. Dimitrov, 'Ovarian Function in Women Having Professional Contact with Metallic Mercury', *Akusherstroi Ginekologiya*, Vol. 13, No. 1, 1974, pp. 29–34

O. N. Syrovadko, 'Working Conditions and Health Status of Women Handling Organosilicon Varnishes Containing Toluene', *Gigiena Truda I Professional 'Nye Zabolevaniya*, 12 (1977), pp. 15–19

O. N. Syrovadko and Z. V. Malysheva, 'Work Conditions and their Influence on Some Specific Functions of Women Engaged in the Manufacture of Enamel-Insulated Wires', *Gigiena Truda I Professional 'Nye Zabolevaniya*, 4 (1977), pp. 25–8

p. 75 'Alcohol Can Damage Unfertilised Eggs', *New Scientist*, 24 March 1983, p. 801. (This drew on papers in the *Journal of Embryology and Experimental Morphology*, Vol. 71, p. 139, and *Nature*, Vol. 302, p. 258)

p. 76 R. P. Knill-Jones, Barbara J. Newman, and Alastair A. Spence, 'Anaesthetic Practice and Pregnancy: Controlled Survey of Male Anaesthetists in the United Kingdom', *The Lancet*, 25 October 1975, pp. 807–9. See also R. P. Knill-Jones, L. V. Rodrigues, D. D. Moir and A. A. Spence, *The Lancet*, i, 1972, p. 1326

p. 77 P. J. Tomlin, 'Health Problems of Anaesthetists and Their Families in the West Midlands', *British Medical Journal*, 1, 1979, pp. 779–84
Letters to the *British Medical Journal*, from Alastair Spence and R. P. Knill-Jones (28 April 1979, p. 1144); Professor Richard Doll (21 April 1979, p. 1078); P. J. Tomlin (12 May 1979, pp. 1280–81)

p. 78 K. Hemminki et al., 'Spontaneous Abortions by Occupation and Social Class in Finland', *International Journal of Epidemiology*, Vol 9, No. 2, 1980, pp. 149–53. See also other papers reviewed by Barlow and Sullivan, op. cit., pp. 32–4
K. Hemminki et al., 'Spontaneous Abortions among Female Chemical Workers in Finland, *International Archives of Occupational and Environmental Health*, Vol. 45, 1980, pp. 123–6

p. 80 Joyce Egginton, *Bitter Harvest*, Secker & Warburg, 1980

p. 81 T. F. Jackson and F. L. Halbert, 'A Toxic Syndrome Associated with the Feeding of Polybrominated Biphenyl-Contaminated Protein Concentrate to Dairy Cattle', *Journal of the American Veterinary Medical Association*, Vol. 165, 1974, pp. 487–9
Joyce Egginton, op. cit., pp. 14–15

p. 82 Joyce Egginton, op. cit., p. 323
Geoffrey Lean, Roger Kerr and Tony Heath, '"Chemicals Killed Our Cattle," Say Farmers', *Observer*, 26 February 1984, p. 6

p. 84 'Child Brain Tumours Tied to Parents' Jobs', *International Herald Tribune*, 4 July 1981, p. 9

p. 85 Oliver Gillie, 'Drugs Taken in Pregnancy Linked to Cancer', *Sunday Times*, 13 September 1981

4: THE PLACENTA BETRAYED

p. 89 Geraldine Youcha, 'Life Before Birth', *Science Digest*, December 1982, pp. 46–53

p. 90 'Twin Vanishes During Pregnancy', *Science Digest*, December 1982, p. 92

p. 91 Thomas Verny and John Kelly, 'The Secret Life of the Unborn Child', Sphere Books, 1981/Summit Books, 1981

Peter Beaconsfield, George Birdwood and Rebecca Beaconsfield, 'The Placenta', *Scientific American*, Vol. 243, No. 2, August 1980, pp. 94–102. See also *Placenta: The Largest Human Biopsy*, ed. R. Beaconsfield and G. Birdwood, Pergamon Press, 1982

p. 98 'The Effect of Environmental Pollutants on Human Reproduction', *Environmental Science & Technology*, Vol. 15, No. 6, June 1981, pp. 626–40

p. 99 J. M. Tesh, 'The Unborn Child: How Well is it Protected?', pp. 139–48, *International Safety Evaluation: Proceedings of a Life Science Research Symposium*, held in Tokyo and Osaka, 7 and 9 March 1978

John R. Holum, '*Topics and Terms in Environmental Problems*', John Wiley & Sons/Wiley Interscience 1977, pp. 633–4

p. 101 Helen B. Taussig, 'The Thalidomide Syndrome', *Scientific American*, Vol. 207, No. 2, August 1962, pp. 29–35

p. 102 *Sunday Times* 'Insight' Team, *Suffer the Children*, André Deutsch, 1979

p. 107 *Report of the Secretary's Commission on Pesticides and Their Relationship to Environmental Health* (the Mrak Report), Parts I and II, US Department of Health, Education and Welfare, Government Printing Office, December 1969, pp. 655–77

p. 108 'The Effect of Environmental Pollutants on Human Reproduction', *Environmental Science & Technology*, Vol. 15, No. 6, June 1981, pp. 626–40

p. 114 Michael R. Moore, 'Lead Exposure and Water Plumbo-solvency', in *Lead Versus Health*, ed. M. Rutter and R. Russell Jones, John Wiley & Sons, 1983, pp. 79–106

5: A MUTANT'S INHERITANCE

p. 120 *Identifying and Estimating the Genetic Impact of Chemical Mutagens*, Committee on Chemical Environmental Mutagens, Board on Toxicology and Environmental Health Hazards, Commission on Life Sciences, and National Research Council, National Academy Press, Washington, DC, 1983, p. 233

p. 121 Debora MacKenzie, 'Secret Tests Say Thalidomide is Mutagenic', *New Scientist*, 18 August 1983, p. 457

p. 123 Donald Clive, 'Human Germ-Cell Mutagenesis – a Subject of Study Without a Subject to Study', *Trends in Biochemical Sciences*, March 1983, pp. 111–12

p. 124 *Living with Radiation*, National Radiological Protection Board, 1981

p. 126 *Guidelines for the Testing of Chemicals for Mutagenicity*, Committee on Mutagenicity of Chemicals in Food, Consumer Products and the Environment, Department of Health and Social Security, Report on Health and Social Subjects 24, HMSO, London, 1981

p. 129 'Chemicals and Genetic Damage', *Nature*, Vol. 301, 24 February 1983, p. 653

6: THE VANISHING THRESHOLD

p. 141 'A Farewell to Regulation', *Fortune*, 19 September 1983, pp. 49 and 52

p. 143 'Reagan's America: The Battle of the Budget', *ENDS Report* 75, June 1981, pp. 10–13

p. 144 'Caligula's EPA Horses', *New York Times*, re-run in *International Herald Tribune*, 28 July 1983
'Watt Future for the Environment?' *ENDS Report* 76, July 1981, pp. 8–10

p. 146 Andy Pasztor, 'Cleaning Up the EPA: Ruckelshaus to Tackle an Agency Mired in Suspicion and Inactivity', *Wall Street Journal*, 2 May 1983

p. 147 John Elkington, *The Ecology of Tomorrow's World: Industry's Environments, Environment's Industries*, Associated Business Press, 1980, particularly 'Nature's Laws', pp. 74–102
Expenditure Estimates Relating to Pollution Control in Germany for the Period to 1980, Battelle Institute, September 1975

p. 151 Des Wilson, 'Do We Need an Environmental Protection Agency in Britain?', *Friends of the Earth Supporters' Newsletter*, Spring 1983, p. 20

p. 152 'The European Commission: Assessing the Environmental Performance of EEC States', *ENDS Report* 78, July 1981, pp. 12–14

p. 155 Fred Pearce, 'Toxic Waste: The Cowboys are Back in Business', *New Scientist*, 11 March 1982, p. 628
Christopher Joyce, 'US Steps Up Trade in Toxic Wastes', *New Scientist*, 11 August 1983, p. 391

p. 156 'Massive Toxic Waste Dump Found Beneath Dutch Housing Estate', *European Chemical News*, 15 November 1982, p. 22
'Greens Demand Hoechst Spends Dividend on Antipollution', *European Chemical News*, 20 June 1983, p. 18

p. 159 *Pollution 1990: The Environmental Implications of Britain's Changing Industrial Structure and Technologies*, a report for the Department of the Environment's Central Directorate on Environmental Pollution, published by Environmental Data Services, London, 1981

p. 164 *Lead in the Environment*, Royal Commission on Environmental Pollution, Ninth Report, HMSO, London, 1983. See also 'How the Royal Commission Swung the Case Against Lead in Petrol', *ENDS Report* 99, April 1983, pp. 9–11

7: TESTING TIMES

p. 168 Nancy Heneson, 'Heads it Causes Cancer, Tails it Doesn't', *New Scientist*, 5 May 1983, p. 275

p. 169 *Occupational Safety and Health: A Du Pont View*, E. I. du Pont de Nemours & Co., Inc., Wilmington, Delaware, 1980

p. 172 The LSR material is drawn from interviews; from *Advances in the Detection of Congenital Malformation*, in the Proceedings of the 5th Conference of the European Teratology Society, 20–23 September 1976, ed. E. B. van Julsingha, J. M. Tesh and G. M. Fava: and from *International Safety Evaluation*, Proceedings of the LSR Symposium held at Tokyo and Osaka, 7 and 9 March, 1978

p. 174 H. Sjostrom and R. Nilsson, *Thalidomide and the Power of the Drug Companies*, Penguin Books 1972, particularly pp. 171–6

p. 175 Sam Shuster, 'Realistic Therapy for the Drugs Industry', *Guardian*, 21 March 1983, p. 8

p. 176 John Elkington, *The Ecology of Tomorrow's World: Industry's Environment, Environment's Industries*, Associated Business Press 1980, particularly 'Vetting Products', pp. 211–38
John Elkington, 'Giving ICI the Green Light', *ICI Magazine*, Summer 1983, pp. 29–34

p. 179 *Guidelines for the Testing of Chemicals for Toxicity*, Committee on Toxicity of Chemicals in Food, Consumer Products and the Environment, Department of Health and Social Security, Report on Health and Social Subjects 27, HMSO, London, 1982

p. 183 *Guidelines for the Testing of Chemicals for Carcinogenicity*, Committee on Carcinogenicity of Chemicals in Food, Consumer Products and the Environment, Department of Health and Social Security, Report on Health and Social Subjects 25, HMSO, London, 1982

p. 184 S. M. Barlow and F. M. Sullivan, *Reproductive Hazards of Industrial Chemicals*, Academic Press, 1982, particularly 'Reproductive Toxicity Testing in Animals', pp. 9–22

p. 187 *Guidelines for the Testing of Chemicals for Mutagenicity*, Committee on Mutagenicity of Chemicals in Food, Consumer Products and the

Environment, Department of Health and Social Security, Report on Health and Social Subjects 24, HMSO, London, 1981

Identifying and Estimating the Genetic Impact of Chemical Mutagens, National Academy Press, 1983, particularly pp. 73–143

p. 190 *Risk Assessment: A Study Group Report*, The Royal Society, London, 1983, particularly 'Laboratory Experiments for Estimation of Biological Risks', pp. 46–75

8: GENE SCREENS

p. 195 S. M. Barlow and F. M. Sullivan, *Reproductive Hazards of Industrial Chemicals*, Academic Press, 1982, pp. 99–100 and 293–4

p. 196 Thomas H. Murray, 'Warning: Screening Workers for Genetic Risk', *Hastings Center Report*, February 1983, pp. 5–8

Editorial, *Chemical Week*, 13 August 1980, p. 5

p. 197 Zsolt Harsanyi and Richard Hutton, *Genetic Prophecy: Beyond the Double Helix*, Bantam Books, 1982, p. 80

T. H. Maugh II, 'Carcinogens in the Workplace: Where to Start Cleaning Up', *Science*, Vol. 197, 1977, pp. 1268–9

p. 198 G. M. Lower, Jr, et al., 'N-acetyltransferase Phenotype and Risk in Urinary Bladder Cancer: Approaches in Molecular Epidemiology, Preliminary Results in Sweden and Denmark', *Environmental Health Perspectives*, 29, 1979, pp. 57–61

p. 199 H. E. Stokinger and L. D. Scheel, 'Hypersusceptibility and Genetic Problems in Occupational Medicine – A Consensus Report', *Journal of Occupational Medicine*, 15, 7 July 1973, pp. 564–73

Herbert E. Stokinger and John T. Mountain, 'Tests for Hypersusceptibility to Hemolytic Chemicals', *Archives of Environmental Health*, 6, April 1963, pp. 57–64

p. 200 'Predictive Identification of Hypersusceptible Individuals', *Journal of Occupational Medicine*, Vol. 24, No. 5, May 1982, pp. 369–74

p. 201 T. J. Ley et al., *New England Journal of Medicine*, Vol. 307, 1982, p. 1469

p. 203 Harsanyi and Hutton, op. cit., pp. 88–9

9: THE TOXIC FRONTIER

p. 206 A. M. MacKinnon, 'Environmental Fears: New Reports Create Climate of "Chemophobia"', *Chemecology*, October 1981, pp. 6–7

p. 207 Jeremy Main, 'The Hazards of Helping Toxic Waste Victims', *Fortune*, 31 October 1983, pp. 158–70

'Toning down the Mediterranean Blues', *The Economist*, 11 June 1983, pp. 69–72

p. 208 Robin McKie, 'Cadmium in the Diet Poses Health Danger', *Observer*, 25 September 1983, p. 5

p. 210 Deirdre Mason, 'Ireland Struggles to Control Pollution', *New Scientist*, 7 April 1983, pp. 14–15

p. 211 Kathleen A. Hughes, 'Chemical Firms Stung by Criticism, Take Lead in Safer Waste Disposal', *Wall Street Journal*, 12 July 1983
'Pollution is on Tap in Silicon Valley', *New Scientist*, 21 July 1983, p. 180. See also Sylvia Collier, Will Elsworth-Jones and Christopher Hird, 'The World's Cleanest Industry Can Damage Your Health', *Sunday Times*, 31 July 1983, p. 17

p. 213 Debora MacKenzie, 'Hamburg Faces Dioxin in the Wind', *New Scientist*, 26 July 1984, pp. 8–9
'Dioxin Hysteria', *Wall Street Journal*, 1 June 1983, p. 6

p. 216 Jeremy Main, 'Dow Versus the Dioxin Monster', *Fortune*, 30 May 1983, pp. 83–91. See also Carla Rappoport, 'Dow Learns to Cope with its Critics', *Financial Times*, 3 October 1983, p. 10

p. 219 'Dow Corning: The Case for Deregulating Organosilicons', *ENDS Report* 106, November 1983, pp. 9–11

p. 221 'Mice Deaths Sound Alarm at Love Canal', *New Scientist*, 29 September 1983, p. 916

p. 222 *Statistics on Experiments on Living Animals*, Advisory Committee on Animal Experiments, HMSO, London, 1983
Nancy Hereson, 'Loophole May Allow Trade in African Chimps', *New Scientist*, 20 October 1983, p. 165

p. 224 'Human Placentas Can Test Drugs Safely', *New Scientist*, 16 August 1984, p. 20

p. 225 Natalie Angier, 'The Electronic Guinea Pig', *Discover*, September 1983, pp. 76–80
Report of the FRAME Toxicity Committee, Fund for the Replacement of Animals in Medical Experiments, Nottingham, February 1983

p. 227 'Drugs to Treat Acne Blamed for Brain Deformities in Babies', *New Scientist*, 18 August 1983, p. 458

p. 228 Moyra Bremner, 'How Drugs Can Turn to Poison', *Sunday Times*, 2 October 1983, p. 13

p. 229 *Risk Assessment: A Study Group Report*, The Royal Society, London, 1983
'Tobacco Affects Chromosomes', *New Scientist*, 15 September 1983, p. 766. Article based on paper by Jennie Kline et al., *American Journal of Human Genetics*, Vol. 35, p. 421

p. 230 'Is Cassava at the Root of Birth Defects?', *New Scientist*, 18 February 1982, p. 437. Article based on paper in *Teratology*, Vol. 24, p. 289
David Weir and Mark Schapiro, *Circle of Poison*, Institute for Food and

Development, 2588 Mission, San Francisco, California 94110, USA

p. 231 Toby Moore, 'Poison Threat in Fresh Fruit and Veg', *Sunday Times*, 5 August 1984, p. 1

David Bull, *A Growing Problem: Pesticides and the Third World Poor*, Oxfam, Oxford, 1982

p. 233 Debora MacKenzie, 'Ignorance was Seveso's Real Disaster', *New Scientist*, 29 September 1983, p. 918

p. 235 Eric Silver, 'Child's Cry Epitomises Bhopal's Nightmare', *Guardian*, 2 February 1985, p. 7

p. 236 Ronald Alsop, 'New Breed of Environmental Activists Wage Fight Against Dumping of Hazardous Wastes', *Wall Street Journal*, 20 April 1983

INDEX

biocides, 31, 46, 48–9, 51, 58, 65, 88, 115–16, 216–19 (*see also* pesticides *and under individual compounds*)
biodegradation, 34
Biodynamics, 172
Bionetics, 172
Bioresearch, 172
biotransformation in placenta, 108
birth control pill, *see* contraceptives, health effects of
birth defects, 18–21, 49, 67, 88, 99, 100–18, 212–13, 214, 226–7, 229, 230, 234, 235 (*see also* teratogens, teratology); genetic aspects, 119–40; superstitions about, 100
birth weight, 88, 112
Black Report, 26–7
Black, Sir Douglas, 26–7
Black, Dr John, 23
Black Du Pont Employees Association, 193
Blake, David, 122
blastocyst, 56, 76, 93, 96. 98, 112
Bliss, Russell, 214–15
Board on Toxicology and Environmental Health Hazards, 14, 120
Boehringer Ingelheim, 10, 213
books, in environmental monitoring, 28
BP, 156
Bradman, Godfrey, 163
brain tumours, 84
brain vulnerability, 99, 113, 161
Brazil, 20–21, 218–19, 234–5
breast milk, contamination of, 58, 65, 70, 79, 80, 86
Bristol-Myers, 224
British Agrochemicals Association, 232
British Medical Association, 231
British Nuclear Fuels Ltd, 25
bronchitis, 18, 196–7
Brooks, Charles, 211
Brown, Governor Jerry, 150
bubble concept, 149
Budetti, Dr Peter, 18
Bunge, Dr Raymond, 51
Burford, Anne, 144–7, 207
Burroughs Wellcome, 123, 139
Bush, Vice President George, 141
butachlor, 167
Butler, Professor Neville, 112
butylated hydroxy anisole, 45
butylated hydroxy toluene, 45

cadmium, 36, 111, 114, 157, 164, 208
caffeine, 54–5, 112
Calandra, Dr Joseph, 167
California Institute of Technology (Caltech), 14, 17, 40–44
Campaign for Lead-Free Air (CLEAR), 163–5
Canada, 145, 148, 167

cancer, 21, 25, 27, 69, 77, 83, 120, 128, 138–9, 183–4, 194–5, 198–9, 202, 213, 215, 221, 226–7, 231, 234; bladder, 197, 198; childhood, 84–5, 125; fish, 23; liver, 125; lung, 22; vaginal, 85, 110–11
Cantlon, Dr John, 149
captan, 116
carbon disulphide, 199
carbonless copy paper, health effects of, 30
carbon monoxide, 67, 111
carbon tetrachloride, 67, 170
carboxyhaemoglobin, 112
carcinogens (*see also* cancer), 11, 21, 23, 27, 83, 120, 168, 170–71, 182–4, 189, 226; transplacental, 83, 117, 231
Carson, Rachel, 46–7, 65, 115, 177, 206–8, 232
Carter, President, 141–7 *passim*, 226
cassava, 230
cataract mutation test, 188
caustic soda, 159–60
Centers for Disease Control, 111, 119, 207, 213, 234
cerebral palsy, 113
Cetrulo, Dr Curtis, 111
Chemagro Corporation, 166
Chemical Manufacturers Association, 211
chemical mutagens, 126–40, *passim*
Chemie Grünenthal, 100–106, 174
Chemie Linz, 213
chemophobia, 206–7
Chesapeake Bay, 211
Chisso production plant, *see* Minamata disaster
Chittam, Dr Brock, 82
chloracne, 214
chlor-alkali production, 209
chlordane, 80
chlordecone, *see* Kepone
chlordifluoromethane, 117
chlorinated butadienes, 23
chlorinated hydrocarbons, 40, 46, 64 (*see also under* biocides *and* individual compounds)
2-chlormethylnapthene, 221
chlorobromuron, 167
chloroform, 117
chlorophenols, 115
chloroprene, 73, 74, 117
chocolate, 112
chorion, 94
chorionic gonadotrophin, 96
Christian, John, 221
chromic acid, 196
chromium, 157, 208
chromosomes, 131–40, 188–9, 194, 229; abnormalities, 49, 56, 75, 188–189, 194 (*see also* Chapter 5)
chronic toxicity testing, 182–91